Gloria Thomas be[...] after working as an actre[...] uch as Patrick Lichfield an[...] specialises in working with children and continues to work as a personal trainer. Gloria is currently a regular contributor to a number of magazines and has recently taken part in a major series of features for the *Mail on Sunday* and is a member of *Zest Magazine*'s fitness advisory panel.

She has also presented a series of video presentations for *Cosmopolitan*, is a spokesperson for Fit Kids UK and is co-presenter with Liz Earle of a forthcoming GMTV health and fitness video.

To Anne Douse,
from your loving daughter

Also available in Orion paperback

AROUSING AROMAS
Kay Cooper

EAT SAFELY
Janet Wright

HEALTH SPA AT HOME
Josephine Fairley

JUICE UP YOUR ENERGY LEVELS
Lesley Waters

SPRING CLEAN YOUR SYSTEM
Jane Garton

APPLES & PEARS

GLORIA THOMAS

ORION

An Orion Paperback
First published in Great Britain in 1998 by
Orion Books Ltd,
Orion House, 5 Upper St Martin's Lane,
London WC2H 9EA

Always consult your doctor first if you have any medical conditions –
such as injuries, diabetes, pregnancy, heart problems, obesity, asthma –
that may affect your ability to participate in exercise.

A CIP catalogue record for this book
is available from the British Library.

ISBN: 0 75281 604 7

Printed and bound in Great Britain by
The Guernsey Press Co. Ltd, Guernsey

CONTENTS

INTRODUCTION 1

CHAPTER ONE
Your Body Type 5

CHAPTER TWO
Storing and Burning Fat 21

CHAPTER THREE
The Muscles 38

CHAPTER FOUR
Stretching and Suppleness 53

CHAPTER FIVE
Posture 59

CHAPTER SIX
Five Steps to Commitment and Success 69

CHAPTER SEVEN
The Warm-up 75

CHAPTER EIGHT
General Exercises 80

CHAPTER NINE
Core Exercises for Each Body Type 91

CHAPTER TEN
Developing a Personal Programme 104

CHAPTER ELEVEN
You Are What You Eat 116

CHAPTER TWELVE
A Healthy Mind 132

BIBLIOGRAPHY
AND ACKNOWLEDGEMENTS 138

INTRODUCTION

'I ndividual' is the key word when it comes to the *Apples and Pears* fitness programme. We are all different, unique in every way: shape, size and form. We each have our own likes and dislikes, good and bad habits. That individuality expands to activity and physical fitness. Exercise means different things to different people. For some people, exercise is simply how far or how fast you can run. For others, it means general health gains to combat heart disease, diabetes or osteoporosis. But for many people exercise is about having the perfect body.

One of the assumptions made about exercise in the past was that we are all the same. General exercise programmes were given, and while many people

an exercise programme specific to the individual's needs

certainly became much fitter and achieved all sorts of health benefits, others dropped out because the exercise they were doing was not specific enough to help them maximise their particular assets. But now, with the boom of personal training in the 90s, awareness has grown of the importance of making an exercise programme specific to the individual's needs.

I started off my fitness career using the premises of a little nursery school off the Wandsworth Bridge Road in Fulham, London. I had two clients, both housewives with children. Each was a completely different shape. One was a classic English pear. The other was a stocky-looking lady with all her body fat carried around her middle, who could be described as having an apple shape. Both were unhappy with their physique. Neither had ever exercised before and each believed that if she did, she would become super-slim, just like the models on the front covers of glossy magazines. I had to explain that they would never be wafer-thin because their basic body types wouldn't allow it. I also explained to them (having first-hand experience because I modelled for many years) that the majority of models were unfit, ate unhealthily and puffed endless cigarettes. Models and not great role models!

Models are lucky enough to be born with good bone structure, regular proportions and long limbs. But being underweight, as many models are, can be as unhealthy as being overweight, predisposing you to problems such as irregular periods and an increased risk of osteoporosis. Problems come for models, like anyone else, at around the age of thirty, when nature takes over. The metabolism starts to slow down and muscles start to lose their tone. After this age a model relies on excellent lighting and a clever make-up artist. The point I was making to my two ladies was that we are all made differently and whether you are two or seventy-two, genetics plays the most important role in determining body shape. There is nothing we can do about it. My ladies recognised that they had to change their mindset, and to accept themselves as they are. They could still look fantastic by making the most of the assets they had.

From the nursery school in Fulham I built up a very broad client base: from local housewives to celebrities, from two ex-Miss Worlds who are now mothers of three, to authors and some very aristocratic titled people. I also worked at an exclusive health club, giving body-shaping classes and personal training, and I specialised in children's fitness. I learned that no one is happy with the shape they have, be they housewife or aristocrat. Everybody wants to change something about themselves. So I set about finding ways of helping people to be the best that they can be within their type.

METABOLIC BODY TYPING

My research first took me back to the three classifications of body types: endomorph, mesomorph and ectomorph. But there are many subdominant types within these three. These classifications did not completely answer my questions. So I was most excited to hear that modern nutritional science had come up with a concept called 'metabolic body typing', which broadens the classifications from three body types to four, and bases them on hormonal and hereditary factors. Dr Elliot Abravenel's work (see Bibliography) furnished me with sound knowledge. From there, I was inspired to help my clients and to explore further.

The Apples and Pears fitness programme works on sculpting the body by reproportioning it: reducing the areas that need to look slimmer and building the areas that need to look bigger. I started to give my clients a better understanding of how their body worked and to make their exercise programmes individual to their type.

The end results were more balanced, more shapely, fitter bodies with better body alignment, and the new inner confidence that comes with having a body to be proud of.

I have had complete success with my clients, and the knowledge I shared with them I now pass on to you.

The Apples and Pears fitness programme works on sculpting the body by reproportioning it: reducing the areas that need to look slimmer and building the areas that need to look bigger

CHAPTER ONE

Your Body Type

The key to the new you is finding out which of the four body shapes you fit into. Remember your body shape is governed by your proportions, not by your height and weight. You could be short and stocky, or medium or tall and stocky. You could be short and thin, or tall and thin. You could have a high weight for your stature, but that does not necessarily mean a stocky build: you might be overweight. Similarly a low weight for stature may mean you are undernourished.

By the age of two you can see a basic body type forming. Between three and four, and seven and ten, small increases of fatness and development of muscle tissue appears with growth spurts. Hormones influence

> *By the age of sixteen your fat cells are laid down, influenced by genetics and lifestyle*

your adolescent shape, and by the age of sixteen your fat cells are laid down, influenced by genetics and lifestyle. (The more active you are as a child, the more you benefit later in life.) By your late teens your adult body shape is established. It may be a combination of one or two types, but you will still lean towards one type. At the end of this section, complete the questionnaire so that you are clear about your predominant shape.

THE G-TYPE

This is the classic English pear-shape, who is most likely to be short or medium in height, with narrow shoulders, a small waist and wide hips.

We call her the G-type because her dominant gland is the gonads, the organs producing the female sex hormone oestrogen. This hormone causes fat to accumulate around the breasts, hips, thighs and buttocks.

'Child-rearing hips' would be the best way to describe the G-type. She's built to survive a famine: she stores extra energy to feed her baby in the fat cells around her hips and thighs, and this fat layer also protects her reproductive organs. Breastfed babies consume large amounts of their mother's calories in the first six to eight months of life and nature safeguards these energy supplies in the hips and thighs of the mother. As the G-type gets older, if she is inactive, her metabolism will become sluggish and

> *The G-type is feminine and curvaceous*

when she becomes overweight the excesses will accumulate on the hip, thigh and breast area. This is called lower-level obesity, because it is predominately below the waist. Because the dominant hormone for the G-type is oestrogen, various health issues may arise from excess oestrogen, such as heavy menstrual bleeding. Overall the G-type is feminine and curvaceous with 'tapered' fingers, shins, ankles, wrists and forearms. She is built for endurance rather than power.

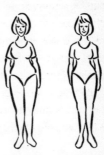

The G-type shape

The good news for G-types is that it is less hazardous to your health to carry weight around your hips and thighs. It is stored there for a sound biological reason. Unfortunately this is not the case with abdominal fat.

CASE STUDY: JESSIE

Jessie was a delightful Irish client with an eight-month-old baby. She was a classic pear, with wide hips and a droopy bottom covered with excess fat and dimples. She had narrow shoulders that had developed a rounded posture through breastfeeding. Jessie's BMI (see page 30) was 26, which meant that she was overweight.

Jessie was permanently exhausted because her baby kept her awake at night. She was breastfeeding and had developed tight pectoral muscles and overstretched back muscles, with resulting aches and pains around her shoulder area. The knock-on effect of her tiredness meant that Jessie was too exhausted to cook and relied on take-aways, especially curries that were full of spices and cream! The birth of the baby had been fairly traumatic and Jessie's aim was to get fit for the next one so that her labour might be easier. She had also lost confidence in herself. She still wore baggy maternity clothes and she wanted a new image. She particularly hated the extreme of her wide hips and narrow shoulders, and wanted a more balanced look.

As Jessie was completely sedentary and she was tired and still breastfeeding, my aim was to develop her exercise programme over a long period of time. I started her off on a light aerobic walking programme, with postural exercises to combat the round-shoulder problem. I also advised her to cut out the spicy foods and to ensure that her diet was low in fat and high in complex carbohydrates, fruit and vegetables. At this stage I had to be her motivation, because she had a tendency to want to give up.

I was determined to encourage her to develop an exercise habit.

After a few weeks I increased her aerobic activity so that she was now outside walking twice a week and inside exercising with a home video once a week. I slowly and progressively added exercises for all her body parts, including core G-type exercises to start shaping her upper body.

After a few weeks more, Jessie seemed to come alive again. She found she had more energy for her household tasks and for the baby and she began to feel good about herself. She began to notice changes taking place in her body. There were fewer dimples on her hips, thighs and bottom and her posture was improving enormously. To use her own words, her shoulders had opened up.

By ten weeks Jessie had reached a base level of fitness and performed her exercises with good technique. By this stage she had stopped breastfeeding and was less tired, so she was able to concentrate on working a little harder. I introduced weights into her programme for her upper body and focused on building up strength and shape in her shoulders. Jessie's aerobic activities increased in frequency as well as duration. As well as losing her excess weight, Jessie's legs became stronger and more toned and her bottom began to lift. Her body mass index shifted from 26 to 24. Jessie was thrilled with her new shape.

THE A-TYPE

The A-type has a more athletic build, with a strong-looking skeletal frame and firm muscular limbs. The shoulders are wide and the neck, chest and waist have a 'thick'-look. The hands are squarish in shape with tubular fingers. The hips are smaller than the shoulders, creating a triangular shape when this body type is lean. These women are masculine in their shape, with powerful buttocks and thighs with muscle fibres that generally respond well to exercise and sport. A-types make good athletes.

> **A-types make good athletes**

On the whole this body type has more muscle mass than fat tissue unless she is overweight and unfit. If the A-type puts on weight, it is generally down to poor lifestyle habits and inactivity, and fat is deposited on the upper part of the body producing a thicker trunk, waist, arms, shoulders and abdomen. In middle age and especially after menopause, she puts on weight more easily, which can cause health problems such as cardiovascular disease and diabetes, and of course apple-shaped obesity. There is evidence that people with excessive abdominal girth have high levels of low-density lipoprotein, a more destructive form of fat carried in the blood.

The A-type is so called because her dominant glands are the adrenals. The adrenals produce the hormones cortisol and adrenaline and the male hormone androgen, which gives her that strong masculine look, energy and strength. These hormones are anabolic, which means they are responsible for building up body tissue. When the A-type becomes overweight through eating the wrong foods and inactivity, her body fat increases and so do the levels of oestrogen and androgens. This can create an imbalance, making the chemical process in the body work even more inefficiently. The result is that metabolism slows down and more weight is gained.

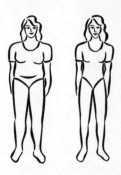

The A-type shape

CASE STUDY: NICOLA

Nicola was an attractive, sophisticated woman in her mid-thirties. I first met her at the exclusive health club where I worked. I used to turn up to take my class and there she would be, gazing wistfully into the studio where the classes were taking place. I often tried to encourage her to go in and try. But she would refuse, saying she was too fat and ungainly and that she would feel stupid.

Nicky's body had interesting proportions. She had a very powerful build with wide shoulders, a thick waist and powerful thighs and buttocks. She carried most of her weight around her middle, which gave her a pot-bellied look and an arched back. Nicky also had excess weight on her shoulders, the back of her arms and her breasts. When I first met Nicky her BMI (see page 30) was 27, her blood pressure was high and she was bordering on obesity. She was also depressed because she was having fertility treatment that wasn't working, and as a result was comfort-eating on large meals with red meat and snacking on salty food.

Nicky's natural competitive instinct made her yearn to go into the studio and work really hard to burn calories away and get back to her ideal body shape, but her main worry was that a big woman doing aerobics would look ungainly and stupid.

With her doctor's permission, I started Nicky on exercise three times per week that was predominately aerobic, and posture work. There was no point in working on body shaping until she had got rid of the fat that was covering her naturally good shape. We started training in the studio with the blinds down so nobody could see, and we worked on just moving her body to very simple aerobic exercises. I taught her that she could be powerful in her movements. After a while her motor skills improved enormously and her movements became more fluid, linking one into another. I also suggested that she cut down on protein and salty foods and snacking.

Soon the weight was falling off her and her BMI was down to 24.

We focused on postural exercises for her abdominals and back, and worked on the problem areas on her upper body. I started gradually incorporating the exercises from the general toning session, working to 15 repetitions, and her muscles responded beautifully. Soon this wonderful athletic shape started to emerge and Nicky sheepishly confessed that she had once run for Scotland in the 200 metres. Her confidence had returned and the last time I saw her she was leaping up and down in an aerobics class, having the time of her life!

THE P-TYPE

The P-type is thick-set, fairly average to large in size and straight up and down in appearance

This body type has been chubby since childhood. The structure of the P-type is thick-set, fairly average to large in size and straight up and down in appearance. Her shape is hard to define because she is covered in layers of fat. Her shoulders are average to large in size, her hips and buttocks curve outwards, her hands are long with tapered fingers, and her abdomen tends to protrude, making her arch her back, which could give her postural problems later on.

The P-type's movements are generally quite slow and she is inactive with a sluggish metabolism. Her body type sets her up for endurance work, not power or speed. If she becomes overweight, fat is distributed all over her body from her face down to her toes. The P-type will always have a problem with her weight so it is important that she watches her eating habits and exercises regularly.

The dominant gland in the P-type is the pituitary gland, situated at the base of the brain. The pituitary gland plays a major role in metabolism by controlling the production of hormones from the thyroid, adrenals and ovaries. Controlled by the hypothalamus, the pituitary is called the master gland of the body. Certain foods are said to over-stimulate the pituitary, which can result in health problems

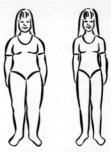

The P-type shape

such as obesity, cardiovascular disease and fluid retention.

For this body type, exercise is a strong stimulant to the hypothalamus and increases the release of all anterior pituitary hormones. It is vital for this body type to stimulate her sluggish circulation and metabolism.

CASE STUDY: MAURICE AND MARINA

My favourite case study is a husband-and-wife team. Maurice and Marina were both P-types. He was 32, 6 feet tall with a BMI (see page 30) of 32, and had had a mild heart attack. She was 30, with a BMI of 30. She had had three children in close succession (they were as big as their parents were). Their proportions were typically those of the P-type: large, thick bone structure, straight-up-and-down look and covered in baby fat from top to toe. She was a smaller version of him, but after three babies her stomach muscles were completely slack, and her upper body posture was damaged by years of breastfeeding.

Their characters, I have to say, were larger than life: the epitome of fat and happy people. I used to love going round to their house because the smell coming out of the kitchen was always mouthwatering. Here, of course, was the root of the problem. Both loved their food and ate huge quantities of it, especially Mexican food, and dishes loaded with cream. Each had a sweet tooth too – disastrous for their body type.

After consulting with their GP, I designed an exercise programme for them. They both needed a programme that was endurance-based so that they could burn calories and tone up their muscles. The difficulty was getting them to do anything. They hated exercise with a passion and every time we got started, they would find an excuse to stop. I despaired of them: they both needed to keep going and their programme was to build to four sessions per week. It seemed an impossible task. I could see dropout looming. One day I put my music tape on to start them exercising. The machine ate my tape! 'Don't worry, I've got some great music,' said Maurice. He got out his favourite salsa music, and that was that. They were off. (A little loud, maybe, for a Saturday morning but who cared?) They shook their stuff, and the house as well. They had so much fun in the first, aerobic, part of the session that they applied themselves more readily to the second part, toning.

I did a lot of postural work with Marina, working on her back, chest and abdominals, and both took part in the general toning sections. Maurice's BMI went down to 29 and Marina's to 28 in the first three months, and then down to 27 and 26, respectively, over a period of time. Each became a good few stones lighter. I was sad when they moved out of London to the country. These people were happy with who they were but recognised they had to do something for their health as well as their shape.

THE T-TYPE

The T-type can be tall, medium or short, with small to average bone structure. On the whole she has long limbs, with long fingers and toes to match. Her shape is likened to that of a supermodel, and she looks very boyish, with slight chest and narrow hips and shoul-

ders. She can also been described as bony, with sticking-out ribs and bony protuberances around the joints. Tall T-types might be round-shouldered, depending on their lifestyle, habits and state of mind.

Her musculature is smaller and frailer than that of the other body types, and her muscle fibres predispose her to excel at endurance sports. She is like a human waste-disposal unit: she can eat huge amount of food without putting on weight thanks to her high metabolism. Like all the body types, as she gets older and because of lifestyle and inactivity, she becomes prone to excess weight, and this is normally distributed around the middle of the body, the upper thighs and abdomen.

The dominant hormonal gland for this body type is the thyroid, at the front of the neck. It releases the thyroid hormone to stimulate oxygen uptake and energy expenditure, and controls the metabolic rate of the body. The T-types are highly strung, sensitive, high achievers, and probably suffer from stress more than the other body types. Under conditions of stress, there is added thyroid and adrenaline release. If the stress keeps up, eventually the thyroid and adrenal glands suffer from exhaustion, which can result in weight gain, or tiredness and lethargy.

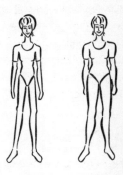

The T-type shape

Women over 35 lose bone mass at 1 per cent per year, and after menopause at 3 to 5 per cent. This body type makes less oestrogen than other types, and if she becomes underweight she will start to produce lower amounts of oestrogen, which will affect her periods and increase the risk of osteoporosis.

CASE STUDY: GLORIA

My last case is me! I am a typical T-type who wants to be curvy and strong. I am a 35-year-old mother of a gorgeous 11-year-old boy. I am a fitness specialist, who focuses on integrating fitness into other people's lifestyles so that they can be the best they can. I often start work with clients at 6 am, and continue to do enormous amounts of physical work throughout the day with mums, celebrities and, of course, my specialist area, children.

My body type is lean with small bones and if I don't exercise I get scrawny and bony-looking. I have a high metabolism and I worry lots about everything. Three years ago my BMI was 17, which is very low. I am 5 foot 6 inches tall and I then weighed just over 7 stone. People subtly suggested that I had an eating disorder. Most annoying, because I eat like a horse! The problem was that although on the whole I ate healthily, I was consuming some foods that overstimulated the thyroid. Coffee and chocolate were my favourites. As a result of this I slept badly, and soon I was not practising what I preached. I became worn out. I needed to make some lifestyle changes or I was going to fade away.

I wrote a prescription to myself. But my first problem was getting to the gym: a wonderful club but I could not justify a 45-minute drive there, 1 hour in the gym and then another 45-minute drive home again. That was time I wanted to spend with my son. Easy really: I joined a local health club, five minutes' walk away, and I started to go there during afternoon cartoon time, when I knew I wouldn't be missed.

I set myself a programme to increase my muscle mass. My base level of fitness was good so I could start with a heavier weight. I was particularly scrawny around my chest, shoulders and arms, so I focused on these areas. I also worked on my legs as my calves needed more shape. I gave myself 30 to 45 minutes, four days a week, working my upper body one day, my lower the next. For cardiovascular work I started taking step classes and circuit training, and I devoted one evening a week to jogging with my son Jamie. I cut down my workload, and I cut out the coffee and chocolate and increased my protein intake. My BMI is now 19 and I am my desired shape.

ESTABLISHING YOUR BODY TYPE

The best way to determine your body type is to have a nice warm bath or shower, and then, still with no clothes

Take a long look at yourself in a full-length mirror

on, take a long look at yourself in a full-length mirror.

If you have problems identifying your shape, think about your childhood. Were you active and sporty? Were you chubby or thin? Think about your structure when you were at your slimmest, rather than focusing on what life has contributed lately. Use the questionnaire which follows to get a clearer idea of your shape. Select the characteristics that apply to you by ticking the box at the side of the page: try to find as many as five. At the end, look up the answers in the table.

☐ **1** I am bigger below the waist than above.

☐ **2** I hold most of my fat around my stomach.

☐ **3** I can eat a lot of food without putting weight on.

☐ **4** My hands and feet are square with fingers that taper only a little.

☐ **5** I have cellulite predominately on my outer thigh and bottom.

☐ **6** I hold most of my fat around the tops of my thighs and middle.

☐ **7** I always had puppy fat as a child.

☐ **8** I have bundles of energy throughout the whole day.

☐ **9** My hands and feet are big with long fingers.

☐ **10** I carry fat all over my body.

☐ **11** I have a strong-looking, muscular frame at my ideal weight.

☐ **12** I hold most of my fat on the bottom half of my body.

☐ **13** My hands and feet are long and slender with tapering fingers and toes.

☐ **14** My structure is thick-set, straight up and down in appearance.

☐ **15** My hands and feet are small with tapered small fingers.

☐ **16** My bones are long and slender with bony protruberances around the joints.

ANSWERS

1 G	5 G	9 P	13T
2 A	6 T	10P	14P
3 T	7 P	11A	15G
4 A	8 A	12G	16T

If you have three or more characteristics of any one body type, this is your dominant type. If you have any less, than you are likely to have a subdominant body type.

QUESTION: If my body is a G-type will I ever look like a T-type?

Sorry, never. Look carefully at your proportions and your body structure. You were not designed to be a T. You have a feminine shape; Marilyn Monroe comes to mind when I think of a G-type. With a combination of aerobic exercise and strength work, you can become slimmer and give your muscles more shape, enhancing that wonderful curvy figure.

QUESTION: Can I make myself into an A-type?

This is the body that we can aspire to because we can all increase our muscle mass and decrease our body fat by slimming down the bits that need slimming down and by building the parts that need to be built. You can train your muscles to be more powerful. You can become closer to this type than any other within your natural ability. The late Princess of Wales trained her body to these athletic proportions.

QUESTION: I'm a combination of two of these body types. What should I do?

This is a subdominant body type. Look carefully at what you have got. Concentrate on aerobic work to slim down or maintain a good body weight and do strength work to shape and strengthen.

WHAT COMES NEXT

The bottom line with your body type is there is very little you can do to change the structure you were born with. A G-type can never be a T-type or vice versa because the basic body shape and the genetic hormones are different. So, with this in mind, start to be positive about your good points and don't get negative about the things that can't be changed. Remember, even the so-called 'perfect' people are never happy with what they've got.

The common denominator with all body types is that inactivity and bad lifestyle habits distort a naturally good shape. If you put on excess weight over the years or fail to use your muscles, you will suddenly find that you are untoned and have aches and pains and postural problems. The key to success with the Apples and Pears fitness programme is to accept the shape that you are born with. You cannot change the structure of your body, but you can use the tools from this book to help you achieve the possible dream of the perfect body shape within your type.

Now that you have established your body type, it's time to get a basic understanding of the components that will help you to build a base level of fitness.

CHAPTER TWO

Storing and Burning Fat

One of the key ingredients to success in the Apples and Pears fitness programme is aerobic exercise. Aerobic exercise plays an important role in body shaping: it exercises the heart and lungs and burns fat. Aerobic means 'with oxygen'. Aerobic exercise consists, therefore, of long continuous movements using the major muscle groups to make the body demand a greater amount of oxygen. It is not only important for body shaping, it is also the basis of a healthy lifestyle in which your body is enabled to cope with the stresses and strains of everyday life.

The major muscle used in aerobic exercise is the heart, which works continuously to pump blood and supply oxygen and nutrients to your muscles and organs. Evidence suggests that there is a lower incidence of heart disease among those who are involved in physical activity, so it is crucial for all four body types to exercise this most important muscle. The lungs are an important part of aerobic work too. Together the work of the heart and lungs comprises what is called cardiovascular activity.

As you begin to exercise, your heart rate increases, delivering blood rich in oxygen, hormones and nutrients to the vital organs and the working muscles of the body. Having delivered its load of nutrients, the blood flows back through the system carrying waste products for elimination.

The more you move your muscles in exercise, the harder the heart has to work to pump blood to give them energy to perform. This pumping action strengthens the heart as well as providing the muscles with energy for performance, and over a period of weeks your heart will start to respond by becoming fitter, pushing out more blood and lowering the rate it beats at rest. For body shaping, the better the whole system works, the more efficiently you will burn calories.

THE FAT-BURNING SYSTEM

To burn calories to lose weight, you need to stimulate your metabolism, or the rate at which you burn energy. Your metabolic rate controls your body weight because it determines how many calories you use to keep your body and your brain going.

Body composition
Your metabolism is affected by your body composition (or lean body mass, which includes bones, muscles and organs, and fat mass). Muscle is metabolically active even at rest, while fat is considerably less so. Therefore, the more muscle you have, the more calories you will burn. Men generally have a faster metabolism than women because they have more muscle mass.

Your height and weight affect the rate at which you burn energy. A taller person burns more calories than a shorter person: a tall T-type compared to a short G-type, for example. A person who is muscular, like the A-type, burns more calories than someone like the P-type, who has a higher proportion of fat and a slower metabolism.

Age
Age affects your metabolism. Your metabolic rate peaks at the age of twenty and declines thereafter. At around thirty you start to lose muscle mass and increase your body fat. If you behave like a couch potato, then as you get older and your metabolism slows down you will gain weight. However, if you regularly exer-

cise with strength and aerobic work, and eat the appropriate food for your type, your metabolism won't change dramatically.

FINDING YOUR METABOLIC RATE

To find your Basal Metabolic Rate (BMR), or to get an idea of how many calories you burn at rest, which includes the beating of the heart, breathing and maintenance of body temperature, you can do a simple equation. Then you can work out how many calories you take in and how much you may expend through exercise (see the activity chart on page 37), which will allow you to lose, maintain or gain body weight.

You may need a calculator for the equation.

Multiply your weight in pounds by 11. Alternatively, multiply your weight by 10; then add your weight again once. For example, if you weigh 130lb:

130 x 10 = 1,300
1,300 + 130 = 1,430

then your BMR is 1,430 calories per day. Reduce the figure by 2 per cent

> *A person in their thirties requires 2 per cent fewer calories than the calculated figure, and a person in their sixties 8 per cent fewer*

for each decade after age twenty. A person in their thirties requires 2 per cent fewer calories than the calculated figure, and a person in their sixties 8 per cent fewer.

THE ROLE OF HORMONES

Each body type has it own unique metabolic rate, governed by the four major glands – gonads, adrenals, thyroid and pituitary

– which secrete hormones into the system. The performance of the glands is affected by the food we eat: of which more later.

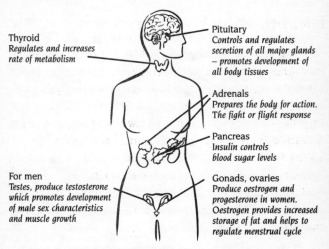

Thyroid
Regulates and increases rate of metabolism

Pituitary
Controls and regulates secretion of all major glands – promotes development of all body tissues

Adrenals
Prepares the body for action. The fight or flight response

Pancreas
Insulin controls blood sugar levels

For men
Testes, produce testosterone which promotes development of male sex characteristics and muscle growth

Gonads, ovaries
Produce oestrogen and progesterone in women. Oestrogen provides increased storage of fat and helps to regulate menstrual cycle

Major locations of Endocrine Glands

The **gonads** are the glands that produce the female sex hormones oestrogen and progesterone, and the male hormone testosterone. Progesterone produced in the ovaries is made from cholesterol, which is made up from the carbohydrates and fats we eat. Progesterone has special functions in preparing the body for pregnancy.

Oestrogens are a group of hormones primarily produced in the ovaries. They control fat distribution on a woman's body. Oestrogen levels vary through life with age, menopausal status and menstruation.

The **adrenals** produce the powerful hormones cortisol and adrenaline as well as the male hormone androgen which makes this body type look masculine. They assist in the conversion in the liver of glucose to glycogen, which is later distributed to all the cells of the body. These powerful hormones control the formation of both muscle and fat, and they increase the mobilisation of free fatty acids, making them a more available energy source. Adrenaline is the hormone that prepares you for action.

Another essential hormone secreted by the adrenals is aldosterone, which causes sodium retention and potassium excretion by the kidneys. We need aldosterone to live.

The **thyroid** gland is the metabolic gland of the body. Responsible for the performance of oxidation in the metabolism, the thyroid secretes hormones into the bloodstream and increases oxygen consumption. The thyroid works to burn food in the tissues and control the flow of glycogen from the liver into the blood. Thyroid hormones are described as calorigenic, because they determine the rate at which the body burns food.

The **pituitary** is the master gland, releasing a number of hormones into the bloodstream. These hormones are involved in the activity of more than one gland, including the adrenals, thyroid and gonads. The pituitary releases the growth hormone, which promotes muscle growth and stimulates fat metabolism. Growth hormone levels are elevated during aerobic exercise and remain elevated after exercise.

BODY FAT

Body-fat distribution is inherited. If one of your parents is overweight, there is a greater chance that you, without loving care and attention, will also pile on the pounds. So take a good look at your biological parents, if you can: they are a good guide of what to do, or what not to do, as the case may be.

Fat makes up a percentage of body weight and is stored all over the body. Each fat cell contains fats, hormones, nutrients and oxygen, all set to be metabolised to give off energy. We store it under the skin, in the skeletal muscles and around the internal organs. We need fat. However, the body can accumulate endless amounts of it, stored in fat cells when not being used. When a person gains weight, fat cells fill up and increase in size. When weight is lost, the fat cells release fat and reduce.

The hormones in a woman's body mean she has more fat than a man. This hormonal influence encourages fat to be distributed in different parts of the body at different times in her life cycle. As body fat increases, so does the production of hormones in the fat cells. A good diet and exercise are essential in reducing body fat.

THE G-TYPE

Our G-type's dominant hormone oestrogen causes fat to be deposited around the reproductive areas of hips, thighs, bottom and breasts. Unluckily for the G-type, fat can easily be stored in this area, but it is difficult to shift because nature put it there to reserve energy for nursing. G-types are also prone to an uneven and lumpy appearance in their hip and thigh area because of the hormonally active fat tissue. This is called cellulite. Aerobic exercise will not only increase general fitness and balance hormone levels for this body type, it will also help to trim body fat around the hip and thigh area, reducing the lumps and bumps of cellulite to reveal the G-type's wonderfully feminine shape.

QUESTION: I am a G-type and I have just gone through menopause. I seem to be accumulating weight around my tummy. Why is this?

After menopause, the hormone levels of oestrogen start to

fall, which results in the change of fat distribution from your hips and thighs to your tummy.

THE A-TYPE

If the A-type becomes overweight, fat accumulates in the upper body, particularly around the waist, breasts, neck, shoulders and the backs of the arms. The excess weight caused by bad diet stimulates the dominant adrenal gland to secrete cortisol and androgens. These hormones are anabolic, which means they are responsible for building up body tissue. When this body type becomes obese, health is at risk, because this type of overweight is associated with cardiovascular disease, diabetes and high blood pressure.

The A-type should have a good low-fat diet and do regular aerobic exercise to maintain a healthy body weight. The good news for the A-type is that abdominal fat is easier to shift than hip and thigh fat.

QUESTION: Can I lose weight from just one place with exercise?

When you lose weight through exercise, fat is taken from stores throughout the body. You cannot draw it from one place. You can, however, spot-tone to tighten up individual areas.

THE T-TYPE

The dominant hormone for the T-type is the thyroid, which supplies her with a metabolism that is fast and efficient. This body type may be the envy of all the others because she eats like a horse and never puts weight on. The T-type appears to have endless staying power but what she may not realise is that the thyroid works in bursts and can become exhausted if it is not rested.

When the T-type feels tired, she stimulates her thyroid with coffee, chocolate and sugar. This can overstimulate the thyroid and the adrenals, and cause them to function less efficiently. Then the T-type's metabolism slows down and fatigue weight-gain occurs around the tops of her thighs and on the abdominal area.

For this body type, a healthy-eating plan is essential in order to strengthen and balance the thyroid hormones, not only to reduce excess body fat but also to combat the up-and-down metabolism.

QUESTION: I am a T-type and have never had a problem with weight gain, but recently I have started getting dimples around my thighs. What is this?

What you have is cellulite, another name for subcutaneous fat. It has been suggested that a hormonal imbalance within the fat cells causes this cottage-cheese effect on hips, thighs and other areas of the body. It could also be attributed to a woman's skin becoming thinner as she gets older, while the connective tissue that builds chambers around the areas where fat is stored becomes stronger. When the fat cells become full, the walls remain firm and fat protrudes over the top. This, combined with the thinning of the skin, results in cellulite. While it may never go away completely, you can improve the appearance of problem areas with aerobic and toning exercise, and of course a balanced diet.

THE P-TYPE

Lastly, our P-types, whose dominant gland is the pituitary. The pituitary governs the activity of the thyroid and the adrenals and has control of the sex glands. The metabolism dominated by the pituitary glands does not affect any one area of the body more than another so this type has an even distribution of fat. When metabolism is sluggish, weight accumulates all over. Although people with this body type tend not to aspire to physical fitness, it is extremely important that they do aerobic exercise to combat their slow metabolism and prevent unwanted weight gain.

QUESTION: I am a P-type who hates exercise. To lose weight can I go on a crash diet rather than exercise?

Yes, but you will probably find that initially you lose mainly fluid and muscle mass. Your metabolism will slow down to preserve energy and once you resume normal eating habits you may find that you will pile the pounds back on – and possibly more than you lost – because your metabolism is slower. When you lose weight through crash dieting, your muscles look untoned and slack. A healthy, low-fat eating plan combined with a mixed regime of aerobic and strength exercise will burn calories and tone your muscles at the same time.

IDEAL WEIGHT: FINDING YOUR BODY MASS INDEX

Ideal weight is difficult to define because everyone is different. Take two people of same height and stature: one probably weighs more than the other. You might assume that the heavier one is the fatter one. However, it may be that the heavier of the two exercises regularly. With exercise, muscle becomes denser and is likely to weigh more than fat.

Your ideal weight is the weight at which you look and feel your best. Bearing this in mind, it is possible to give an indication of what is an average weight for your height. The most scientific way is to find your Body Mass Index. You need to work in metric to find this. Divide your weight in kilograms by the square of your height in metres.

For example:

Weight: 60 kilos

Height: 5 foot 5 inches, or 1.65 metres

1.65 x 1.65 = 2.7225

$$\frac{60}{2.7225} = BMI\ 22$$

You should aim to keep your BMI between 19 and 25. Less than 17 is underweight. Between 25 and 29 is overweight and greater than 29 is obese.

CALORIE BURNING

What is the best way to burn calories? Answer: Get moving! Exercise that is continuous and rhythmic and uses the major muscles of the body is best. How long you exercise and how hard you work are instrumental in calorie-burning. These in turn depend on your fitness levels and the energy systems you use.

How the body burns calories

The muscles use two systems of calorie burning. One is the aerobic system, where the fuel is predominately fat, broken down in the presence of oxygen. Water and carbon dioxide are the waste products. The aerobic system is capable of generating large amounts of energy because both fat and oxygen are available in abundance. Together they work to burn calories: a crucial part, of course, of a weight-loss programme.

The other is the anaerobic system, which produces energy without depending on oxygen. Its source of fuel is carbohydrate, which is not as high in calories as fat, and which is available for immediate use in the muscle. The waste product is lactic acid, which you feel as you tire quickly.

The anaerobic system kicks in when the intensity of an activity increases to a point where the aerobic system cannot supply enough oxygen to meet the body's energy demands. This sort of energy is used by athletes to increase their capacity for speed and power. Sprinting is a good example, as is a fast ball-game like squash. Think of the last time you had to sprint for a bus and were gasping for breath as a result.

You could use both systems to burn calories, because ultimately what matters is the quantity, not the quality, of calories you burn. If you are a complete beginner to exercise, you will find that initially you may burn carbohydrate and tire quickly because your aerobic system is not yet able to cope with the energy demands placed on it. As fat is the more efficient fuel source, I suggest that a complete beginner works aerobically at a low to moderate intensity for about 20 to 30 minutes at a time. This puts less stress on the body than working at a high intensity. A fitter individual may work harder by increasing the intensity of the workout.

I do not advise anaerobic training to the totally inactive, but if you have a good base level of fitness, then have a go. Anaerobic activities include hockey, squash, netball (all of which involve short hard bursts of action), and short sharp bursts of fast cycling, swimming, running.

If you persevere with aerobic exercise, you will see that, as you become fitter, your body learns to metabolise fat better. The more you exercise, the more the oxygen sent to the

As you become fitter, your body learns to metabolise fat better

working muscles increases, which in turn improves the process of calorie burning. Your system becomes more efficient at burning fat and you lose weight.

AEROBIC EXERCISE

There are many different ways of working aerobically. The following are recommended activities for calorie-burning. The chart on page 37 gives you calorie expenditure for different activities, influenced by your body weight (in kilos). Now that you know your BMR (see page 24), you can add to this the additional calories you expend during activities, and compare the result against what you take in as food. This should help you either to lose or to maintain your body weight.

One point to remember. Don't expect miracles immediately. It took a long time to put on all those excess pounds and they will not disappear overnight. Losing fat the right way takes time, and setting up lifestyle patterns and creating new habits is important. Studies have shown that fat should come off the body at a rate of 2 pounds (about 1 kilogram) per week, depending on the amount of fat there is to lose and also on your diet and activity levels. With this in mind, think slim thoughts – not thin ones – and go for it!

> *Losing fat the right way takes time, and to set up lifestyle patterns and create new habits is important*

AEROBIC ACTIVITIES

These exercises are good for every body type: fast walking, jogging, step aerobics, tennis, badminton, cycling, swimming, treadmill, stair master, rowing, cross-country skiing and aerobic dance. Indeed, when it comes to dance, any type of vigorous dancing will do: country, Latin, rock 'n' roll, line – all great fun even if you have two left feet. A caution to body types G and P. If you choose to ride a stationary bike, make sure the resistance on the machine is low so that you are not building up the muscles in your thighs and bottom. Your aim is to slim and trim, not build up in these areas.

Tips
* Try to combine different activities to prevent both boredom and repetitive stress on the joints.
* Wear comfortable footwear that supports the ankle and heel.
* Drink plenty of fluid before, during and after exercise to replace fluids lost from the body.

Aerobic composite training
A great way of adding variety to your workout is by composite training. Combine different activities into your exercise session to reach your goal: for example, 10 minutes of fast walking, 10 minutes of stepping, 10 minutes of dancing. This is great calorie-burning activity. Even though you are working the same muscle groups, you are working different fibres within those muscles.

Interval training
This is where exercise is split into high-intensity activities with low-intensity periods in between. For example: 3 minutes of hard cycling on a stationary bike at a target heart rate (see below) of 60–70 per cent, followed by 2 minutes of gentle cycling where the body is still working but at zero load. Another variation is to combine walking and running.

Circuit training
This type of training is used for the all-round development of fitness. A combination of machines or stations is set up so that participants can move from one to the other. Circuits can offer strength work, or aerobic work, or a combination of the two.

FREQUENCY AND DURATION

For weight loss, three to five bouts of aerobic activity a week is recommended. It is very important, however, that you start as you mean to go on, and that you do not set yourself goals so high that you end up dropping out. Do what you realistically can. If that is twice a week, that's fine, although the process will then take much longer. Having a rest day is also important, to allow muscles to recover and to minimise the risks of overtraining.

For fat-busting you need to think of building up to at least 20 minutes of aerobic exercise after your warm-up. Intermediate exercisers can either

> *For fat-busting you need to think of building up to at least 20 minutes of aerobic exercise after your warm-up*

work harder for that length of time or increase the time to 30 minutes. Over a period of time substantial improvements will be made. Once you have reached the correct intensity during your workout, you need to sustain the pace. To find out your correct exercise intensity you need to monitor your heart rate.

Intensity: *monitoring your heart rate*
Your heart rate will give you an idea of the intensity you are working at. Using a special watch that measures the heartbeat is the most accurate way I have discovered of working out heart rate: especially effective for clients who complain that they are working too hard when I know they are not!

Taking your pulse is a reasonably accurate alternative to using a watch. You need a piece of paper and pen to record your results. On the thumb-side of your left wrist, find your pulse using the two forefingers from your right hand. Take your pulse for 15 seconds then multiply by 4 to get a 60-second pulse reading. Do this first thing in the morning when you have just got out of bed to determine your resting pulse. As you become fitter, you will find that the number of beats decreases.

Having recorded your resting pulse, you now want to work out the intensity that your heart is going to work at when you exercise. First you need to find your maximum heart rate: to do this, take your age away from 220. Your target heart rate for exercise will be 55 to 85 per cent of your maximum heart rate, depending on how hard you are going to work. (The range is broad because of the different levels of fitness. The fitter you become, the higher the appropriate exercise intensity.) I recommend starting at 60 per cent. As you progress and become fitter, you can increase your target heart rate.

Suppose you are 30 and you want to work at 60 per cent maximum heart rate. Your maximum heart rate is 190 (30 from 220), of which 60 per cent is 114: your target heart rate will be 114 beats per minute during exercise. To determine your heart rate during exercise, at an appropriate moment take your pulse again, counting how many beats in 15 seconds then multiplying by 4. You should be at your target heart rate. Otherwise adjust your workout to increase or decrease your intensity.

Your recovery rate is how long it takes your heart to return to normal after exercise, a good indicator of your fitness level. To establish your recovery rate, wait 2 minutes after exercising, then take your pulse again. Do a 15-second count and multiply by 4. The fitter you are, the quicker your heart rate and breathing will return to normal.

If all this is a bit complicated, a much easier way of monitoring your heart rate is through the talk test. If during exercise you can sing the national anthem you are not working hard enough. If you cannot speak at all because you are too out of breath, you are working too hard. You want to aim for a breathy conversation.

Overload

Each individual has an exercise level they feel comfortable at. However, in order to gain fitness benefits and lose weight, you need to be challenged. As you progress, you will be able to work longer and harder and you will need to increase the challenge. This can be done by boosting the intensity, lengthening the amount of time or increasing the number of exercise days per week. You need to aim for overload: it is only at overload that you start to progress.

You need to be aware of the dangers of overtraining, however. Working too hard can lead to injuries and over-fatigue because mind and body become exhausted. Symptoms of overtraining include breathlessness, high heart rate, dizziness and extreme fatigue. With all this in mind, you are now well equipped to start burning calories. Have fun.

CALORIES USED IN 30 MINUTES OF ACTIVITY

Body weight in kilos	50kg	55kg	60kg	65kg	70kg	75kg
Walking:						
@ 20-minute/mile	105	115	126	136	147	157
@ 16-minute/mile	120	132	144	156	168	180
Swimming:						
Slow crawl	192	211	230	250	269	288
Fast crawl	240	259	283	307	331	355
Running:						
@ 9-minute/mile	290	318	347	376	405	434
@ 6-minute/mile	378	416	454	491	529	567
Aerobics	154	170	185	200	216	251
Active dancing	252	277	302	328	353	378
Cycling	150	165	180	195	210	225
Circuit training	174	191	201	226	244	261
Volleyball	75	83	90	98	105	112
Badminton	90	99	108	117	126	135
Tennis	165	181	198	214	231	248

Activity lasting 30 minutes

CHAPTER THREE

The Muscles

F or body shaping, we need to look at muscles. You can tone your muscles to make yourself look slimmer, or you can increase your muscle mass and decrease your body fat to increase the definition of your figure. You can also, depending on genetics and fibre type, train your muscles to look bigger. Before we go on to different training methods, it helps to have a base understanding of how your muscles work.

The body has more than 600 muscles. They come in three types: smooth muscle, which lines the arteries and blood vessels; cardiac muscle; and

> *You can tone your muscles to make yourself look slimmer*

the muscle we are most interested in, skeletal muscle. Muscles are surrounded and attached by connective tissue, which merges with the muscle fibres. Without it, the muscle would tear quickly.

Muscles come in different shapes and sizes. Big muscles, such those in the legs and bottom, carry out powerful movements such as walking, running and jumping, whereas small muscles like those in fingers and hands are responsible for more refined and precise movements.

Skeletal muscles are the body's support system. Without them you would collapse in a heap. They are attached to joints, which act as levers. Movement is brought about through the motor nerves attached to these muscles, whose job it is, acting under instructions from the brain, to stimulate the fibres so that the muscle contracts. When a muscle contracts, it pulls on the bone to make it, and you, move.

The diagram below will give you a good idea of the position of your muscles, and which muscles we will be working in the Apples and Pears fitness programme.

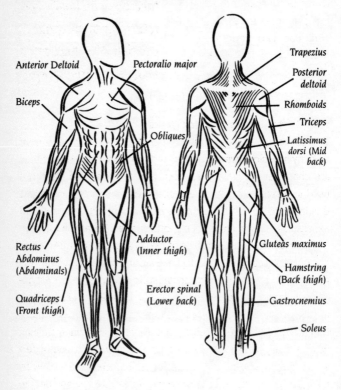

Anterior Deltoid

Biceps

Pectoralio major

Obliques

Trapezius

Posterior deltoid

Rhomboids

Triceps

Latissimus dorsi (Mid back)

Rectus Abdominus (Abdominals)

Adductor (Inner thigh)

Gluteas maximus

Quadriceps (Front thigh)

Erector spinal (Lower back)

Hamstring (Back thigh)

Gastrocnemius

Soleus

The muscles

Training your muscles

To gain maximum benefit in training your muscles, you need to carry out each exercise slowly. The more slowly you perform an exercise, the greater the tension. The general rule in fitness training is to take twice as long when returning to starting position as it took to make the initial move: for example, in a bicep curl, use two counts to bring the muscle slowly up then take it back down in four counts.

> *The general rule in fitness training is to take twice as long when returning to starting position as it took to make the initial move*

Slow-twitch and fast-twitch fibres

Your muscles contain two fibre types that are determined from an early age: slow-twitch and fast-twitch fibres. Fast-twitch fibres are characterised by a quick response to stimulation and are used in explosive bursts of exercise such as sprinting or weight training. Slow-twitch fibres have a slower contraction speed and are associated with endurance sports such as marathon running.

There are no reliable studies of body types and distribution of fibres. Most people are said to have around 50-50. However, it is generally understood that muscular sporty people like our A-type in peak form have a predominance of fast-twitch fibres. Their muscles respond more quickly to exercise so they look more toned. This body type needs to be aware of this when training against heavy resistance, in order not to bulk up. It is also understood that T-types are built more for endurance and are likely to have a predominance of slow-twitch fibres. Overweight people have a higher proportion of slow-twitch fibres, and our G-types and P-types are more likely to come into this category.

To discover which muscle-fibre type you are, think back to school or when you were more active. Were you a fast runner? Did you excel at explosive sports, did you prefer activities that were endurance-based, or were you generally unsporty?

Knowing the shape, position and fibre-type of your muscles and understanding how they work will give you a clear idea of your limits and capabilities, enabling you to perform your exercises with greater control and knowledge.

HOW HORMONES AFFECT MUSCLES

Hormones affect the growth and development of body tissues and so influence the changes that take place in our muscles when we exercise. The endocrine system sends hormones into the blood to travel as messengers throughout the body and to specific areas called target cells.

Target cells have hormone receptors. The interaction between receptors and hormones has been compared to a lock (receptor) and key (hormone) system, in which only the correct key can unlock an action in the cells. When we exercise, we increase blood concentrations of hormones, which interact with receptors.

All body types release the same hormones, though proportions differ with body type. During activity, hormone release changes, which is a further benefit of exercise.

GROWTH HORMONE

For the P-type, exercise is important because it elevates levels of growth hormone both during activities and after. Growth hormone, one of the most well-known hormones, is involved in the growth and repair of muscle and other tissues in the body. Secreted from the pituitary gland, the highest levels are given out at night during sleep. It has been suggested that growth hormone influences the chemical process in muscle development, increasing muscle mass and playing an active role in metabolism.

QUESTION: Does this mean that I will bulk up my muscles through strength training?

How big you will become when you exercise and the shape of your muscles are both largely genetic. It is highly unlikely that a woman will ever look like a body builder because women have less muscle mass than men, and of course less testosterone. So unless she spends hours each day in a gym or takes stimulants, a woman will not get body-builder muscles.

If you are genetically disposed to bulking, you need to be aware of your body-fat levels. Working with heavy weights for strength will change the size and shape of your muscles. If you are covered in layers of fat and you strength train, then you are going to look bigger. The answer is to lose the fat through aerobic exercise so that the muscles look well defined underneath. You then need to focus on strength-training at the correct intensity for your type.

THYROID

T-types are lean and rangy because of their dominant hormone, the thyroid. The function of the thyroid hormones is to set the rate of the chemical reactions that occur in the body. They have a direct effect on tissue metabolism and have the power to increase basal metabolism by up to 100 per cent.

Thyroid hormones are calorigenic: they stimulate oxygen uptake and energy expenditure. With exercise the release of thyroid increases, boosting metabolism and oxygen consumption. Strength training is an ideal way for the T-type to work out because although it increases the metabolism it

> *Strength training is an ideal way for the T-type to work out*

burns fewer calories than aerobic exercise does. The T-type, burning up calories on her own without any help, does not need to undertake a great deal of aerobic exercise for body shaping. Strength training will also give the muscles shape, which will give a more curvy appearance.

ADRENALS

The A-type is strong and powerful with an abundance of energy and staying power. The adrenals, the dominant gland in this type, produce powerful hormones such as cortisol and the male hormone androgens. These hormones are anabolic: they are responsible for building up tissue.

The adrenals also produce the two catecholamine hormones, norepinephrine and epinephrine. These hormones prepare you for fight or flight action. They increase force and energy availability in the muscle. Muscular activity increases the catecholamine release, which in turn increases the breakdown of energy in the muscles and the liver. The adrenals are more important than any other hormone for the expression of strength, hence the A-type's powerful build.

GONADS

The G-type's dominant glands are the gonads, which are the reproductive glands of the body: the ovaries and the testes. The ovaries secrete oestrogen which promotes the development of the female sex characteristics and provides the increased storage of fat which the G-type tends to accumulate around her hips and thighs. Oestrogen also assists in regulating the female cycle. Exercise has a positive effect on balancing oestrogen levels before, during and after the monthly cycle.

The testes secrete androgens, of which testosterone is the most commonly known. Testosterone helps in the development of male sex characteristics and in skeletal muscle growth. Testosterone is responsible in part for muscle hypertrophy (enlargement). Both men and women have testosterone in their bodies but men have at least ten times more, which is why they not only have more muscle but also have the potential to build more muscle than women do.

> *Exercise has a positive effect on balancing oestrogen levels before, during and after the monthly cycle*

STRENGTH VS ENDURANCE

Muscle is active tissue using a large amount of energy even at rest. With age and inactivity, muscle starts to decrease in strength and size. With a decrease in muscle mass, the metabolic rate starts to slow down, which in turn can lead to an increase in body fat, influencing our appearance as well as our physical capacity.

Strength exercise – working against resistance – increases the metabolism by stimulating the muscles to become stronger and larger so that more calories are burned. In this way the muscle loss that normally accompanies ageing is slowed down or even reversed. Working against resistance will help you to maintain or build muscle throughout middle and later life so that the musculo-skeletal system is strongly balanced and tightened. This promotes good posture, helps prevents injury and, of course, helps to fight off the degenerative conditions such as osteoporosis and arthritis that come with age.

There are two very different expressions of strength. The first defines strength as the maximum amount of force a muscle produces in order to overcome a resistance. The second defines strength as muscular endurance, the muscles' ability to perform repeated muscular actions over a period of time. Muscular endurance is, of course, increased through gains of muscular strength, so the two are related.

In exercise we look at strength as the ability to apply progressive force to stimulate muscles into growing and becoming stronger (the first definition of strength). Strength training means exercising individual or specific groups of muscles against progressive resistance. When a muscle works against resistance it is stimulated into growing, increasing the size and strength of muscle fibres and resulting in greater physical abilities and a firm, sculpted-looking shape. Strength-training, therefore, plays a major role in enhancing shape by exercising specific individual and group muscles, and can help you to become the shape you have always wanted to be.

Endurance exercise can be aerobic exercise or individual exercises at a low weight with a high rate of repetitions. You can develop endurance by supplying blood to the muscles through repetitive move-

If you haven't achieved your desired shape in the past it may well be that you have trained your muscles wrongly

ments to burn calories and give the muscle a toned look. If you haven't achieved your desired shape in the past it may well be that you have trained your muscles wrongly. You may have worked your muscles too much in one way, going for too much endurance and not enough strength. The important fact you need to remember is that the more resistance you apply to your muscles the more sculpted they will become, while doing endless repetitions of an exercise without, or with little, resistance will not have such an effect on your muscles. The following section looks at body types and our two different training methods.

BODY TYPES AND TRAINING

It is crucial for our four body types to recognise the difference between the two different types of training so that they can develop an understanding of the methods they might use to give them their perfect shape (within their type). They can have a programme that is based predominately on endurance or on strength, or a programme that is a combination of both.

For example, a lean T-type is unlikely to acquire a good body shape if she does predominately endurance work. She will lose weight and tighten up but probably look too thin. To achieve a curvier shape she needs a good all-round strength-training programme to increase muscle mass so that her muscles will look firm and sculpted and therefore more shapely. The T-type needs to work more with strength than endurance.

> *The T-type needs to work more with strength than endurance*

QUESTION: If I work with weights and then give up exercise, will my muscles turn to fat?

Muscle and fat are two different tissues. Fat cannot turn into muscle and vice versa. If you stop exercising, your muscles lose their size and tone. If you continue poor eating habits, the calories you would have burned off in exercise become additional calories that are stored as fat.

The A-type, once she has lost excess body fat, needs to tone or define her muscles. This body type is quite lucky: her muscles are likely to respond to exercise quickly. The A-type can either maintain her good body shape with endurance work to keep body-fat levels low and her muscles toned, or progress to strength work to achieve a more defined and stronger athletic shape. Because this body type responds quickly to exercise, it is important to keep body fat low in order to avoid a 'bulky' look.

QUESTION: Will resistance work make me lose my bust?

Diet and aerobic exercise are most likely to influence fat deposited on your bust. Strength-training will tone up the pectoral muscles around the bust, giving it support and a firmer-looking appearance.

Our G-type needs to determine what she needs from a toning programme. She has a bottom-heavy build with fat accumulating around her hips, thighs and bottom. An endurance programme will help her slim down into a smaller, more toned G-type. Heavy strength work would be inappropriate as she needs to slim down her lower body, not build it up. However, the G-type who feels unproportioned with a narrow upper body and wide lower body, should, once her fitness levels allow it, focus on a good strength-training programme for the upper body so that her shape becomes more curvy and balanced, creating an hour-glass effect.

QUESTION: Should I use heavy or light weights?

It very much depends on your goals. If you are aiming for light toning of your muscles, use light weights. If you are aiming to increase size and definition, then you should use heavier weights. However, I would stress to a beginner whose muscles may not be used to exercise to start off with no weights then to progress to light ones. Build up a base level of fitness and then focus on your goals.

The G-type needs to use heavier weights for the upper body and no weight or very light ones for the lower body exercises.

The P-type's musculature is thick-set and heavy and quite slow to respond to exercise stimulus. She needs to have a predominately endurance-based programme to lose weight and work on good posture by toning and tightening her muscles. Working with heavier resistance will make this body type look bulky, especially if she is overweight to begin with.

QUESTION: How long do I have to keep exercising?

If you stop exercising once you have achieved your desired shape, your muscles will eventually return to the state they were before you exercised. To maintain strength and tone in your muscles you need to work out all your body parts at least once or twice a week, making sure that you work jolly hard when you do.

OVERLOAD

The overload principle applies as much to strength and flexibility work as to cardiovascular fitness (as seen in Chapter 2). In order to achieve a toned look you need to put gradual progressive stress on your muscles. You might start with just ten box press-ups, then when those become easy progress to doing a few more, so that the body adapts to the new challenge placed upon it. To progress and become stronger and firmer you need to apply more force. If you stay at the same level and do not progress, there will be no further increase in strength and tone. If, on the other hand, you find that you are doing more and more repetitions in order to achieve overload, you will increase your endurance rather than your strength, and not get the full benefit out of your training programme.

SETS AND REPS

Resistance-training exercises are performed in sets and reps (repetitions) in order to progress and get the best results in a muscle. Repetitions are the repeated movement of a weight to bring your muscles to fatigue. A set is a group of repetitions. You might, for example, perform 2 sets of 15 reps each. Generally there are two sets to an exercise programme, or even three sets as you become fitter, though you will invariably start with just one set.

To become stronger and more toned, a muscle needs to do at least 8 to 20 repetitions of an exercise, depending on the goals of your body type. If you are a T-type, you want to work at the lower end of scale, focusing more on strength. If you are a P-type, you need to focus on the other end, for endurance. The A-type is in the middle, and the G-type needs to work at the lower end of the scale for her upper body and the upper end for her lower body.

Each body type needs to work to scale, to a point where she cannot do any more. If you find you can easily do more reps then you need to increase the resistance. If you are working to increase muscle definition and size you want to increase the intensity of your workout by adding more resistance to your muscles.

FATIGUE

Muscle fatigue comes in different forms and is generally caused by the effort of the last few repetitions of an exercise. You may find your muscles quivering or weak and unable to perform any more because they have been depleted of energy, or you may get muscle soreness caused by the build-up of a waste product called lactic acid. Lactic acid is generally metabolised by the body and removed at the end of the exercise session or soon after. You may also find you have soreness over the few days following exercise. This is caused by tears in the connective tissues that hold the muscles together, as well as some tearing of the muscle cells.

While it is perfectly normal to feel challenged on those last few repetitions during exercise, you should not feel pain in your joints. Pain in a specific area can turn into a serious injury. If you are so sore and stiff that you have difficulty moving, then you did too much too soon and you need to work less intensely. You may also discover that you are sore in specific parts of the body. If so, you can still work out the 'unsore' areas but you need to monitor the intensity of what you are doing so that technique and posture are not compromised.

> *If you are so sore and stiff that you have difficulty moving, then you did too much too soon and you need to work less intensely*

TECHNIQUE

Any form of exercise can be stressful to the joints if performed incorrectly. Doing too much too soon, being in the wrong posture or putting your body into an unnecessarily stressed position can compromise your technique, which affects the quality and the safety of your workout. By jerking your movements or performing them too quickly you will not be working your muscles through the full range of movement, which can decrease the flexibility in the joints and potentially cause injury. In exercise it is essential to avoid any strain. For a complete beginner it is a good idea to start an exercise without weight or with minimum resistance in order to learn the correct technique, and then to progress slowly. I always believe it helps to talk myself through an exercise and I certainly always use a mirror when I am learning a new exercise. Listen to your body and monitor how you feel.

MUSCLE BALANCING

When you are putting together your training programme you need to choose exercises that will balance all your muscle groups. The function of the muscles is to provide support and stability to the skeleton. Unbalanced muscles can cause postural problems.

The best way to ensure muscular balance in exercise is always to work sets of opposing muscle groups. If you work your biceps, you need to work your triceps. When you have worked your quadriceps (front thigh muscles), you then need to work your hamstrings (back thigh muscles). The personalised training programme at the back of the book will give you a specialised exercise regime, enabling you to balance all your muscle groups.

The exercises in this book are carried out by using free weights as a form of resistance. As well as free weights there are other ways of strengthening muscles in exercise, such as resistance bands, gym machines, and of course body weight. However, free weights, or dumbbells as they are also called, add a lot more variety in exercise, are low in cost and are functionally very good, particularly when it comes to developing joint strength in the wrist, elbows and shoulders. They also allow you to train both sides of the body equally and so can help to identify weaknesses in your muscles, such as when one side is weaker than the other. You can also work a muscle group in more than one way, exercising different muscle fibres and making your workout even more effective.

Dumbbells are either fixed or adjustable. I recommend that you go for the adjustable, so that you can alter your weights as you become stronger.

CHAPTER FOUR

Stretching and Suppleness

*S*uppleness is the final component of fitness in the Apples and Pears programme. Suppleness, or flexibility, is a joint's ability to move freely throughout a full range of motion. A number of factors can limit flexibility, the most common being the inability of the muscles surrounding the joint to stretch to their maximum length. Most people have the ability to move through a greater range of motion than their muscles will generally allow.

The aim of stretching in exercise, and indeed at any time, is to enhance suppleness: to relax and reduce muscle tension and to maintain and increase range of movement. The important thing is to stretch regularly and properly with correct technique.

> *Suppleness, or flexibility, is a joint's ability to move freely throughout a full range of motion*

No one body type is more flexible than another. A lean, skinny person such as our T-type might be more flexible than someone with a heavier, stocky body shape, such as our G-type or P-type, but you could also find a flexible P-type and a totally inflexible T-type. Flexibility is specific to the individual: to her genetic inheritance and lifestyle. Put more simply, flexibility is specific to your level of activity and to your joints.

Tension

Today's stressed lifestyles can make us inflexible: the tension held in the body causes tightness and stiffness in the limbs and joints. We wake to find ourselves in a hunched position, our bodies stiff and tight, particularly around the shoulders, after having slept in the same position all night. We may be conscious of this tension or completely unaware of it. The result is still the same: tight, tense muscles.

When you stretch, you lengthen your muscles to increase movement around your joints. Through stretching, you can work to maintain suppleness or develop flexibility so that your body can work more efficiently. Stretching also reduces tension, relaxing the muscles and promoting relaxation both physically and mentally.

Stretch reflex

The muscles are enhanced by the force and duration of a stretch. The longer you hold a stretch the more you will develop flexibility. To prevent your muscles from overstretching and becoming damaged, a mechanism called the stretch reflex comes into play. This sends signals to the spinal column which returns an order to create a sudden muscular contraction. When muscles are stretched quickly or with jerking, bouncing movements, the reflex contraction will be faster and more forceful, and it is possible that injuries will occur. Always stretch slowly and smoothly.

QUESTION: Will stretching help me to lose weight?

Stretching cannot help you to lose weight. You can increase your circulation, release tension and improve your posture with stretching but it will not enable you to get fat out of a fat cell.

THE IMPORTANCE OF STRETCHING

For all four body types, stretching is an essential part of a fitness programme, not only to prepare the body and increase flexibility, but also to alleviate the muscle bulking that can arise from the short contractions of exercise. Stretching also gives muscles the appearance of being longer and so improves posture and gives a leaner look.

QUESTION: When do I stretch?

Any time, any place! Stretching is best when the body is warm. You need either to be in the correct (warm) environment or to have raised your body temperature such as by marching in place or brisk walking. Stretch before the main activity of your workout to prepare your muscles, and after your workout when the muscles should be really warm and pliable but short and in need of stretching back into line. It is also important to stretch the key muscle groups that you are using. Each body type needs to do the specific stretches for their core exercises as well as the general stretches: these are covered in chapters 8 and 9.

STATIC STRETCHING

The safest and most common method of stretching during an exercise programme is static stretching. Everybody can do it, regardless of ability, age or sex. Indeed, the older you are, the more vital it is to stretch to maintain suppleness. A static stretch is a slow and gradual stretch, without any bouncing or jerking. You hold the stretch for a period of time. As you hold the position, you feel the tension of the stretch in your muscles. When the tension eases, allow your muscles to stretch a little further to maintain or develop flexibility. If you feel any discomfort, ease off.

THE EASY STRETCH

All body types should start with an easy stretch. These are stretches held for a relatively short period of time: 10 to 15 seconds. Take your time getting into the correct position and be aware of where you feel your stretch – it should be in the bulky part of the muscle. Hold the stretch until you feel tension in the muscle, then when the tension disappears stretch a little further. You should never feel pain when you stretch. If you do, you are overstretching or stretching wrongly. Easy stretches in exercise are perhaps best performed at the beginning of an exercise routine to prepare your muscles for the session ahead: see Chapter 7, The Warm-up.

YOGA

Not only is stretching an important part of any exercise programme, it is also a specific form of exercise on its own. In yoga, for example, the postures are stretches that are held for a long period of time, which both stretch and strength the muscles in a different way to ordinary exercise. Yoga is an excellent addition to any exercise programme. It is important, however, to find a class of the correct level. Some of the postures are advanced and the body must be practised to do them: a yoga teacher will advise.

QUESTION: How often do I stretch?

Every time you exercise, and beyond that, as often as you want. Just be aware of the tensions in your body. The American College of Sports Medicine recommends that you stretch at least three times a week in order to maintain and develop flexibility.

DEVELOPMENTAL STRETCH

Each body type should follow the easy stretch at the end of an exercise session with a developmental stretch. During developmental stretching tension is increased to a level beyond the easy stretch and held for a longer period of time to lengthen the muscles after use. Only when you feel the tension releasing in the muscle should you progress further. These stretches are held for 15 to 30 seconds.

QUESTION: Is it possible to overstretch?

Yes. Excessive stretching can cause overstretched ligaments which can lead to joint instability. (Ligaments hold bones together for stability.) Once a ligament becomes over-stretched you may lose the support around the joints. It is important not to force your muscles beyond their capabilities, so stretch only until you feel a gentle tension in your muscles, no strain.

CHAPTER FIVE

Posture

Within your basic body type, the shape of your body is also determined by postural factors. The way that you sit, stand and move around is strongly affected by both your mental and physical state. If you feel happy and good about yourself, you are likely to hold less tension in your body. However, if you are depressed, angry or feeling just plain miserable, you are likely to find tension accumulating in different areas of the body – depending on the individual.

To prove the point, watch people as you go about daily life. Look at your family and friends, be aware of the people around you at the office or supermarket or on the bus or train. Look for the hunched shoul-

> *The way that you sit, stand and move around is strongly affected by both your mental and physical state*

ders, crossed legs, and other tell-tale signs of stress.

In addition to our mental outlook, physical influences affect our posture. Body type has some influence on how we hold ourselves, but allowances must also be made for the individual variations in lifestyle, age, height, body composition and physique. For example, whatever your body type, if you sit daily for hours in a poorly designed chair, strain and tension will accumulate in the neck and shoulders and the middle to lower back, which can result in overstretched, weak back muscles and a rounded stance. Breastfeeding can cause the body to slump forward and chest muscles to tighten, creating a hunched look in the shoulders. Being on your feet all day, being pregnant or wearing high heels can tilt the pelvis and overarch the back. An older woman may have a rounded, humped spine (a dowager's hump), aggravated by the loss of calcium in the bones, which also results in loss of height.

BODY TYPES AND POSTURE

While all our body types are vulnerable to the same postural faults, some characteristics are particular to each type. If an A-type becomes obese by putting weight on around her middle and upper body, it is quite likely that she may get a bad back caused by strain. Without the support of strong abdominal muscles and chest and back muscles, the extra weight gradually causes a forward tilt of the pelvis, resulting in tension in the lower back, unbalanced upper body musculature and round shoulders.

Tall T-types who are shy or awkward about their height, or who work in such a way that they lean with shoulders hunched forward, could well develop a stooped posture or round shoulders, which will then cause muscular imbalance in the chest and back muscles.

Our bottom-heavy G-type, carrying excess weight around her lower half, can develop poor tone in the buttock, abdominal and lower back muscles.

The P-type, who has a tendency to put on weight all over, could be prone to a top-heavy posture and a rounded back, because of the excess stress across the neck, shoulders and chest, and also to an overarched lower back, caused by the excess strain around her middle and lower body.

At first bad posture merely looks ugly and sloppy, but if left uncorrected it can cause strain on the joints and ligaments which leads to aches and pains. These affect your overall health and wellbeing.

> High heels cause postural problems by upsetting body alignment and shortening the calves. If you love high heels, try to wear them only for best.

> If you work at a desk, make sure the chair and desk are at the right height for you so that you can sit and work without straining any part of the body. This will help to prevent you developing round shoulders.

> If your job causes you to sit or stoop for hours, stop and stretch every half an hour to take away muscular tension.

> Divide your shopping between both hands instead of carrying it all in one, or better still, use a back pack so that the weight you are carrying is central. Carrying weight regularly in only one hand causes an imbalance around the body: the spine will be affected, and the muscles on one side will become overstretched, while their opposite group becomes tight and bunched.

ASSESS YOUR POSTURE

Ideally, to answer this questionnaire, you need two mirrors so that you can get a good view of yourself both front and side. You can only get a really objective view of yourself if you are naked or in your underwear. Be honest with yourself: it's worth it.

My jaw juts forwards	☐ yes	☐ no
My shoulders are rounded forwards	☐ yes	☐ no
My shoulders are hunched up to my ears	☐ yes	☐ no
My lower back is very hollow	☐ yes	☐ no
My stomach sticks out	☐ yes	☐ no
My knees turn in	☐ yes	☐ no
My knees turn out	☐ yes	☐ no
My feet turn in	☐ yes	☐ no
My feet turn out	☐ yes	☐ no

If you have answered mainly yes to these questions, you need to spend a little time on a daily basis adjusting your posture. You may be surprised to find this difficult and uncomfortable at first. This is because your mind has become used to the adopted posture, and your mind needs training into new habits. But if you make a commitment to be much more aware of how you carry yourself, you will find yourself able gradually to stop bad old habits and create good new ones. Aim to set up a lifestyle pattern of good posture that will look good as well as benefit your health.

Ideal posture should show an upright body with a straight line from your ear through the centre of your shoulder, hip, knee and ankle.

IMPROVING POSTURE

Exercises to improve posture

TRANSVERSE ABDOMINALS

One of the groups of muscles primarily responsible for posture is the abdominal group. Strong abdominals give a firm, flat stomach and support your lower back. The most important abdominal group to start with is the transverse abdominal muscles, which wrap around you like a corset.

These muscles are responsible for support and for protecting the internal organs. If your transverse abdominals are weak, it is likely that at some point your back will be affected.

Spend a few minutes each day doing the following exercise.

Lie on the floor with knees bent and arms by your side. Focus on your breathing, allowing it to be steady and natural. Now shift your attention to your abdominals. Breathe in, and as you breathe out pull your tummy in as tight as you can as if to pull your belly button towards your spine. Hold for 5 seconds and gently release. Repeat this about 10 times or as often as you can until you feel those abdominals working.

SHOULDER SHRUG

This exercise focuses on the trapezius, the triangular muscle across the back of the neck and shoulders. Standing or sitting in an upright position with abdominals pulled in, raise the shoulders up towards your ears and then press them down towards the floor. Do this 8 to 16 times or until your shoulders feel more relaxed and more mobile. You can progress with this exercise by using weights, starting with 3-pound (1.5-kilos) weights and moving up to 5-pound (2.5-kilo) ones.

DEALING WITH POSTURAL FAULTS

Two of the most common postural faults are an exaggerated lumbar lordosis, and kyphosis.

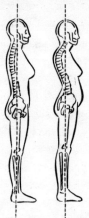

normal posture   *lordosis and kyphosis*

LORDOSIS

Lordosis (an exaggerated inward curve in the lower spine) is linked to tight hip flexors (front hip muscles) and weak abdominal and gluteal (buttock) muscles. People affected by a lordosis are generally those who are on their feet all day, pregnant women, obese people, and women who wear high heels.

Exercises to combat lordosis

HIP FLEXOR STRETCH

This exercise is to stretch out tight hip flexors. You may need the support of a chair or the wall. Stand with your feet together. Put one leg behind you, taking the heel off the ground. Bend your knees. Tuck your pelvis under and hold for 10 to 20 seconds. Do this 10 times.

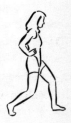

GLUTEAL RAISE

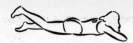

This exercise strengthens the buttock muscles (the gluteals) and the back of the thigh (the hamstring). Lie on your front (you may want to use a cushion under your hip bones for comfort), with hips pressed to the floor. Relax your head in your hands. Keeping the legs straight but not locked, lift and lower each leg alternately. Do this 10 times for each leg, and remember to keep hips square to the floor. As it becomes easy, increase the number of reps.

KYPHOSIS

Kyphosis (curvature of the upper spine) is linked with having tight pectorals, weak upper back musculature and weak abdominals. The people who are most prone to kyphosis are those who spend long periods of time leaning forward, tall people, and people who are top-heavy and who slouch forward.

Exercises to combat kyphosis

FLY

This exercise strengthens the upper back muscles, in particular the rhomboids and posterior deltoids (see diagram on page 40). Use no weights at first, but as you progress gradually add from 1 pound (0.5 kilo) up to 3 pounds (1.5 kilos). You need a bench or the floor (preferably a bench because it allows for a greater range of movement).

Lie face down on the bench with your arms hanging down to the floor (or face down on the floor with your arms by your sides). Take your arms out to the side (at right angles to your body), squeezing your shoulder blades together. Make sure you do not hunch up your shoulders or jerk or bounce, and that you keep your head and neck relaxed. Do this 10 times, increasing the number of reps as it becomes easy.

PECTORAL STRETCH

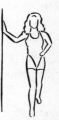

This stretch focuses on the pectoral muscles that become tight with all that slouching forward. Stand next to a support or a wall. Take your inside leg slightly forward and soften your knees. Take the arm nearest to the wall behind you to just below shoulder level. Placing the forearm on the wall, press your body forward until you feel tension in the chest muscles. Hold for 10 seconds. Make sure you don't hunch your shoulders in this position.

It is possible to have both postural problems: an exaggerated lordosis and kyphosis. This is called kyphosis lordosis posture: the head is slightly forward and the upper back is rounded, while the lower back is overarched and the knee joints are slightly hyperextended (locked back). Do the exercises for both lordosis and kyphosis for this.

HOW YOU MOVE

Dynamic or moving posture is as important as static posture because the way you move affects the way you carry and project yourself. If you are happy, you will walk with a spring in your stride, but if you are feeling miserable you are likely to slump, slouch and develop a lazy posture. Bad body alignment – through the foot up into the knees, up the back of the legs into the pelvis and lower back and then into the shoulders, neck and head – is caused by the foot being in the wrong position. The position of the head is also important: where the head leads the rest of the body tends to follow. So make sure you are not jutting your chin forward, but instead tuck it in so that you feel a lengthening at the back of the neck. With the correct posture you can look taller, feel better and move with ease. Try the following exercise

Stand with your back against a wall, touching the wall with head, shoulder blades, buttocks and heels. Hold your abdominals in. As you walk away from the wall, make sure your feet and knees are facing forwards: heels go down first, then roll through to the ball of the foot and toes.

EXERCISE POSTURE

It is essential to start an exercise programme as you mean to go on. Correct exercise posture is of paramount importance: it enables you to work safely but effectively, without tension or strain. A stable base prevents injury and encourages good form and body awareness.

Stand with feet hip-distance apart, knees straight but not locked. Pull your abdominals in and slightly tuck your pelvis under so that your spine is in a neutral position. Lift up through your ribcage and press your shoulders back and down. Relax your chin. Feel the top of your head reaching towards the sky and the whole of your spine lengthening. Breathe naturally and normally.

This posture exercise should be carried out before and during all exercise activities.

CHAPTER SIX

Five Steps to Commitment and Success

By now you should have a clear idea of your body type and an understanding of how the body works through stamina, strength and suppleness. Now you are almost ready to become actively involved in the Apples and Pears fitness programme: a little mental preparation is all that remains.

STEP 1 WORK OUT WHAT YOU WANT

Start by sitting down and working out what it is you want from exercise, however 'plain commonsense' the answers. Writing down your aims, desires and goals will give you clear idea of what you need to focus on and will allow you to feel more committed.

	YES	NO
You are exercising for weight loss	☐	☐
You are exercising to tone muscles	☐	☐
You are exercising to improve posture	☐	☐
You are exercising to improve flexibility	☐	☐
You are exercising to control stress	☐	☐

How many times a week could you commit to exercise?
☐ Once   ☐ Two or three times
☐ Four times   ☐ Five or six times

How long do you think you   When will you exercise?
could realistically spend   ☐ Morning
exercising in each session?   ☐ Late morning
☐ 20 minutes   ☐ Lunchtime
☐ 30 minutes   ☐ Afternoon
☐ 45 minutes   ☐ Evening
☐ more than 45 minutes

If your goals are to lose weight, you need to work aerobically at least three, maybe five times a week. Do the sums and find out your BMR (see page 24). Add up the calories you consume over the period of a week and then add up the calories you need to use up in activity (see the chart on page 37). Remember, if a negative balance is achieved, you will lose weight. If your calorie intake is greater than you use, you will gain weight.

You can also help reach your goals in weight loss as you become fitter by increasing the duration of your exercise, such as from 20 aerobic minutes to 25 or 30, or increasing the intensity of your workout from 60 to 70 or even 80 per cent of your maximum heart rate (see page 36), depending on your

> *Add variety to your exercise regime by walking one day, and dancing, stepping, cycling, rollerblading on others*

fitness level or simply by monitoring how you feel. Add variety to your exercise regime by walking one day, and dancing, swimming, stepping, cycling, rollerblading on others. Use back-up workouts in the form of home exercise videos or your favourite music to dance to. Remember to warm up and cool down properly.

If your aim is largely for muscle toning and reshaping, focus on a strength-training programme of no more than three sessions a week. Remember that muscles need at least a day's rest between sessions to do their work.

Make sure you do the general exercises in Chapter 8 and then the core exercises for your body type from Chapter 9. Introduce the core exercises into your programme one by one.

Don't forget to stretch all the muscle groups you have used for flexibility and posture. Hold the stretches for as long as you comfortably can to lengthen the muscles as far as they can go. You may also choose to incorporate yoga into your programme as an excellent form of stretching. For postural work, use the exercises Chapter 5.

If you want to control stress, then aerobic exercise, strength work and flexibility work are great forms of stress busting. Take a look as well at the relaxation chapter at the end of the book.

You also need to bear in mind that overoptimistic statements – 'I'll be fit and lose two stone in a month' – and 'no pain no gain' philosophies are not advisable. Overdoing it is likely to result in injury and dropout, although of course the less exercise you do the longer it will take to achieve results. However, better to do less and be consistent than to do more and give up after a few months.

STEP 2
FORMALISE YOUR GOALS

Take your plan of long-term goals (from step 1) and break it down into the medium- and short-term goals that make your long-term goal achievable.
Then draw up a contract between you and a friend or member of your family. This will increase your responsibility and commitment to your programme.

CONTRACT OF EXERCISE

I, Gloria Thomas, will undertake to attend all of my scheduled exercise sessions (four times a week) for the next four weeks. The times that I will take my exercises will be Monday, Wednesday, Friday and Saturday at 9 o'clock for one hour, and if for any reason I don't make that time I will give an alternative time so that I will complete my exercises. My helper is Veronica Pieters and she has agreed to prompt me to attend and complete all my sessions. To reward myself at the end of each week that I attend all my sessions I will take myself and my friend to the cinema.

Signed   . . . .

Participant . . . .

Helper   . . . .

Date   . . . .

When you have completed your monthly goal and rewarded yourself and your partner, make up your next month's contract.

STEP 3 KEEP A RECORD

The third step to a committed programme is to keep a record of the changes in your body shape over a period of time. The aim of body-shaping exercises is to maximise assets or minimise faults. Girth measurements are the most valuable way to do this in the home.

Each body type's goals may be different. For example, G-types perhaps aim to increase the shoulder size while slimming down the hips. An overweight A-type may need to monitor the body-fat levels around her bust and abdominals. The P-type will most likely be looking for an overall reduction in size and the T-type may want to increase her measurements all over.

Ask someone to measure you, and try to get the same person to do it each time so that there is consistency in the tension of the tape. Follow the standardised areas as described, make a note of your measurements, and then put them away until it is measuring time again: six weeks or so later.

WHERE TO MEASURE

SHOULDERS	across the widest part
CHEST	at the nipple line during midpoint of normal breath
WAIST	at the narrowest point below the ribs
HIPS	feet together, at maximum protrusion of the buttocks
THIGH	at crotch level
CALF	at widest part or maximum circumference
UPPER ARM	at widest part or maximum circumference

STEP 4 MEDICAL CONDITIONS

Now is a good time to consult your doctor if you have any medical conditions that may affect your ability to participate in exercise.

STEP 5 EQUIP YOURSELF

Lastly, make sure that you are well equipped. You may want to invest in dumbbells (either a set or an adjustable pair), ranging from 3 to 5 pounds (1.5 to 2.5 kilos) in weight. You may need a mat.

Make sure you wear comfortable clothes so that your movements are not obstructed. A supportive bra helps for any aerobic work.

Always have a bottle of water to drink from before, during and after exercise.

CHAPTER SEVEN

The Warm-up

B efore you start exercising, you need to prepare your body by warming up properly. This is a fundamental part of the session. An effective warm-up lasts 5 to 10 minutes. It increases the blood flow, raises the body temperature gradually and loosens the joints, making them less vulnerable to injury.

At the end of the warm-up you need to stretch your muscles to make them pliable and ready for action.

Finally, a good warm-up helps to prepare the brain to focus on the exercise ahead. Start by getting into exercise posture (see page 68).

BREATHING

The breath is the life-force of the body, giving energy to every cell of your being. Many of us have lost the art of breathing properly, and we often use only part of the lungs instead of the whole. Correct breathing focuses the mind and instils discipline and control in the body.

Start to establish a natural, even rhythm. Breathe in through the nose and allow the breath to expand the lungs, ribs and back. Breathe out slowly and easily, letting the ribs fall and without forcing the breath.

THE WARM-UP

Do each warm-up exercise 8 to 10 times.

SHOULDER CIRCLES

In posture position. Circle your shoulders forwards, up, back and down. Keep your movements smooth and controlled.

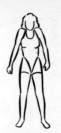

SIDE BENDS

In posture position. Make sure hips stay facing forward, and slightly bend your knees. Pull your abdominals in and gently reach down sideways from side to side.

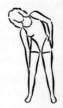

KNEE BENDS

In posture position. Bend your knees in line with your toes for one count and straighten them for one count.
* Make sure you don't lock your knees

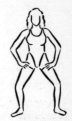

ANKLE CIRCLES

Stand on your right leg with your right knee slightly bent. Tap the left heel and toe on the floor alternating between the two. Change legs.

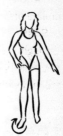

RAISE THE TEMPERATURE

Now you want to raise your body temperature by getting moving. Marching, rhythmical-movement dancing or using an indoor bike or treadmill – if you have one – warm you up effectively. So put on your favourite record and dance, march around the room, or stationary-cycle, for 5 minutes.

STRETCHING

These are lower body stretches, to be used before and after cardiovascular work and for general stretching. For the specific exercises (which come later), I suggest you stretch the muscles of the group you are going to be working both before and afterwards, to prepare them and to promote flexibility. Make sure you hold all stretches for 8 to 10 seconds.

Lower body stretching

CALF STRETCH

Take a step forward with your right leg and bend the right knee. Make sure the left leg is behind the right leg and straight with the heel of the back foot pressed to the floor. Make sure the toes of both feet are facing forward and that a diagonal line runs from the heel of the back foot to the top of your head. Hold the stretch. Now do the other side.

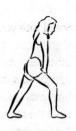

HAMSTRING STRETCH: BACK THIGH

Extend one leg forward and slightly bend the other one. Now placing your hand on the top of your thighs, lean your body weight forward from the hips. Keep your abdominals in and your chest lifted. Feel the stretch in the back of the thigh, not the knee. Hold the stretch. Now do the other side.

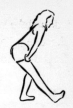

* Make sure you don't lock your knee or arch your back

QUADRICEPS STRETCH: FRONT THIGH

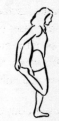

Using a chair or wall for support, shift your weight on to one leg and soften the knee. Bring the heel of the other leg up towards your buttocks, reaching for the ankle and holding it. Tuck your pelvis under. Hold the stretch. Now do the other side.

* Keep your thighs parallel
* Knee should face the floor

ADDUCTOR STRETCH: INNER THIGH

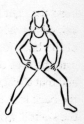

Stand with your feet wide apart, toes pointing slightly out. Bend one knee and extend the other leg, making sure you keep the body upright and hips facing forward. Lower your hips until you feel a stretch in the inner thigh. Hold the stretch. Now do the other side.

* Keep the bent knee in line with the toes

CHAPTER EIGHT

General Exercises

This chapter covers all major muscle groups used in everyday life. These are the foundation exercises that each body type should do to tone and sculpt the body. The core exercises that come in the next chapter are the extras specific to each body type. They can be progressively added to the general exercise section.

Each body type needs to build a base level of fitness with these general exercises, initially working without weights for up to 2 sets of 15 repetitions, concentrating on good posture and technique. When you can do this amount of exercise with ease, progress to light hand-weights and thereafter branch out to the specific needs of your type. The G-type, for example, needs to end up with a programme that allows her to do 10 to 12 repetitions on her upper body and 15 to 20 on her lower body so that the two are balanced. The A-type needs to work to a programme where she is completing 15 reps on each exercise for all-over body toning. The T-type needs to work to 10 to 12 reps to increase her muscle mass, and the P-type 15 to 20 reps for a leaner look.

Remember to warm up, and to spend time stretching at the end of each session to maximise the length that your muscles can go. Remember not to add too many exercises for one body part right from the start.

Remember to warm up, and to spend time stretching at the end of each session to maximise the length that your muscles can go

PRESS-UP: PECTORALS, TRICEPS

On all fours in a box shape on the floor. Knees under hips, hands directly under shoulders with fingers pointing forward. Hold your stomach in tightly so that your back does not hollow, and lean slightly forward so that your body weight is over your arms.

Action
Bending the elbows, push the palm of your hands into the floor. Keeping the body weight over the arms, bring the 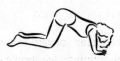 chest towards the floor. Two counts down. Now push through your hands and straighten the elbows without locking them to push your body back into starting position in four counts.

Modification
Move your hands forward about 6 inches (15cm) so that your hips are forward of the knees instead of directly underneath them.

SHOULDER PRESS: DELTOID, TRICEPS, TRAPEZIUS

Sit on a chair or use a bench. Take your dumbbell in each hand at shoulder-width apart. Bend your elbows and bring your dumbbells to shoulder height, palms facing forward.

Action
Breathe out and press the dumbbells straight up above your head for two counts, holding then lowering two counts.

* Keep your back straight: do not arch it by sticking your chest out as you lift your arms
* Start with a low weight; do not try to lift too heavy a dumbbell until you are comfortable with this weight
* Do not lock arms when you extend
* Keep ribs lifted and shoulders down

ONE-ARM ROW: LATS, RHOMBOIDS, BICEPS

Take a step forward with your left leg and bend it in front of you. Your right leg should be straight and behind you. Lean on your left leg with your left arm and hold your abdominals in. Holding a weight in your right hand facing the body, allow the right arm to hang low towards the floor.

Action

Pull the dumbbell towards your ribcage for two counts so that the elbow ends up at shoulder height, and then back for four counts. Make sure the elbow stays close to the waist as you lift.

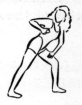

* You can also use a chair bench or some other sturdy object to support yourself
* Make sure you don't grip the weights too tightly

SQUAT: QUADRICEPS, HAMSTRINGS, GLUTEALS

Stand with your feet just outside hip distance apart, toes facing forward, keeping body weight in your heels.

Action

Bend your knees and press your hips out behind you as if about to sit on a chair. Hold your abdominals in and your ribs high to maintain a flat back. Now straighten your legs by pushing up through the heels and squeezing your buttocks. Make sure you don't lock your knees.

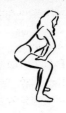

* Shoulders should be in line with your knees and knees should be in line with toes; do not bend your knees more than 90 degrees
* You can increase the intensity of this exercise by holding a weight down by your sides or on your hips

BICEP CURL

Sitting or standing position, upright with abdominals in and chest lifted. Arms hanging by sides with a dumbbell in each hand facing forwards.

Action

Keeping the elbows and shoulders in a fixed position, curl the dumbbells towards your shoulders for two counts, pausing then lowering four counts.

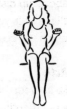

* Back straight * Elbows in
* Shoulders fixed

ABDOMINAL CURL

Lie on your back with knees bent and feet flat on the floor about hip distance apart. Tighten the abdominals in and very slightly tilt your pelvis so that your lower back is flat. Place your left hand behind your head for support and reach out with your right hand towards your knee.

Action

Exhale. Tighten your abdominals and then use them to lift your shoulders off the ground for two counts. Slowly lower two counts, keeping the abdominals in tight.

* Do not pull on your head
* You should not feel strain on your neck
* Do not hold your breath
* Avoid resting your head completely on the floor when you go back to starting position
** Variation 1: with arms crossed over chest
** Variation 2: both hands supporting the side of the head

OBLIQUES

Lie on your back with knees bent and feet flat on the floor about hip distance apart. Tighten the abdominals in and very slightly tilt your pelvis so that your lower back is flat. Place one hand behind your head and the other by your side.

Action

Raise your head and shoulder off the ground, bringing the shoulder toward the opposite knee. Two counts up and slowly back two counts.

* Take care not to roll the hips
* Lead with the shoulder in a diagonal direction
* Do not pull on your head

BACK EXTENSION

Lie on your front and bend your
arms so that palms are on the floor and in line with your shoulders. Keep your hips and feet pressed to the floor and face looking straight down at the floor.

Action
Slowly raise your chest and shoulders off the floor using the muscles of your back, not your arms.
* Only raise as far as comfortable
* Keep feet and hips pressed to floor
* Keep head relaxed
** Variation: place your hands on your buttocks instead
   of on the ground

OUTER THIGH LIFT: ABDUCTOR

Lying on your side with your legs together and your head resting on your arm. Legs should be in line with hips and shoulders. Bring your top hand in front of you to support yourself.

Action
Raise the top leg to shoulder height
and then lower for two counts.

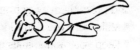

* Make sure your knees and toes are facing forward
* Keep the legs straight but not locked
* Pull your abdominals in to support your back

INNER THIGH LIFT: ADDUCTOR

Lie on your side with both legs together. Now bring the top leg in front of the underneath leg (you may want to put a cushion underneath your knee for comfort and to allow for a greater range of movement) with the knee bent.

Action

Lift the lower leg so that you feel the muscles working in the inner thigh, then gently lower, keeping your heel off the ground.
* Make sure the knee and toes face forward
* Squeeze and tense the inner thigh as you lift
* Keep your heel off the ground

STRETCHES

Hold each stretch 8 to 10 seconds for warm-up and at least 15 to 20 seconds for cool-down. Remember to stretch both sides, where appropriate.

CHEST STRETCH

Sitting or kneeling position with an upright posture and holding the abdominals in. Lift up through the chest. Take your arms behind you and press them away from your back. Hold.
* Make sure you don't lock your arms
* Keep your abdominals pulled in

UPPER BACK STRETCH

Sitting cross-legged on the floor in an upright position. Press your shoulders down and hug yourself, bringing both hands to your shoulder blades. Hold. (You can also do this kneeling or standing.)

* Drop your chin
* Feel your shoulder blades moving apart
* Don't hunch shoulders

BACK STRETCH

Stand about two feet (60cm) away from the arm of your sofa, facing it. Lean forward with hands on the inside of the arm rest. Now bend knees and press hips out 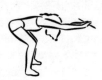 behind you as if about to sit down. Keep your head in line with your spine and make sure you don't bend your knees more than 90 degrees. Hold.

SHOULDER STRETCH

In standing, kneeling or sitting position, gently bring your elbow across your chest towards your opposite shoulder. Use the opposite hand to gently support the elbow. Hold. Now change sides.

* Make sure body faces forward so that you don't become twisted
* Keep shoulders relaxed

QUAD (FRONT THIGH) STRETCH

Lying on your left side, resting your head in the palm of your left hand. Keep the rest of your body straight. Bend your top leg towards your back and, holding your right foot with your right hand between the toes and the ankle joint, gently ease the right heel toward the right buttock, keeping the thighs parallel. Hold. Now change sides.

* You can lie on a towel for comfort

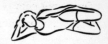

BUTTOCK STRETCH

Sit on the floor with your legs crossed. Extend your arms forward in front of your body. Gently ease forward, placing elbows and hands on the floor. Hold.

ABDOMINAL STRETCH

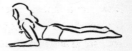

Lie on your front and place your hands flat on the floor in front of you at shoulder level so that elbows are in line with shoulders. Lift the head and shoulders off the floor by pushing up on your hands. Keep hips, elbows and feet on the floor. Hold.

OBLIQUES STRETCH

Lying on your back on the floor with knees bent and arms out at shoulder level. Let your knees drop over to one side, and hold this position. Now change sides.

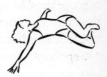

* Keep both feet on the floor
* Keep both shoulders on the floor

LOWER BACK STRETCH

Lying on your back, hug your knees to your chest. Hold.

TRICEPS STRETCH

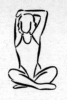

Sitting, kneeling or standing position. Hold a towel in your left hand. Take your left arm over your head, bending the elbow. Reach your right arm up your back towards your left hand and hold on to the other end of the towel or until you feel the stretch in your upper arm. Hold. Now change sides.

OUTER THIGH STRETCH

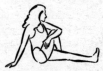

Sit on the floor with your right leg straight in front of you. Bend your left knee and cross it over the right leg. Keep your left hand on the floor. Use the right hand to gently ease the left knee towards you. Hold. Now change sides.
* Keep both buttocks on the ground
* Feel the stretch on the outside of your left thigh

INNER THIGH STRETCH

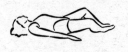

Lie on your back. Bring the soles of your feet together and make a dia- mond shape. Let your knees drop out to the sides. Hold.
* Make sure you hold your abdominals in
* Apply a little pressure with your hands to the inner thigh area to increase the stretch

CHAPTER NINE

Core Exercises
for Each Body Type

THE G-TYPE

The G-type needs to perform lots of aerobic activity to maintain an ideal body weight or lose stubborn unwanted pounds, especially around the hips, thighs and bottom area. I most recommend lots of walking, dancing, aerobics, cycling, swimming. Aim for long duration with low to moderate intensity. (Remember, talk test or pulse monitoring – see page 36.) The G-type needs to avoid high-resistance aerobic work, such as stationary bike, stair masters or stepping machines at a high setting, as this work will give the thighs and bottom a bulky look. Do ensure, however, you do lots of toning for your hips, thighs and bottom.

Once the G-type loses weight she becomes a slimmer G-type. If you are happy with that, then stick to the general exercises. However, if your aim is to balance and shape the upper body, focusing on the muscles of the shoulders, back and chest so that your shape becomes more curvy, then you need first to build a good base level of fitness, working with a weight that allows you to complete 10 to 12 repetitions (not too heavy that you cannot complete 10 to 12 reps, but not so light that you feel little resistance). Then build the core exercises, one at a time, into your general exercise session to ensure your shoulders don't get overworked too soon. Remember to stretch all the muscle groups used. Do not add more than two to three exercises to a body part.

UPRIGHT ROW: TRAPEZIUS, DELTOID, BICEPS

This exercise can be performed in a seated or standing position. The aim is to work the muscles of the upper back. With correct posture, extend your arms down in front of you with dumbbells in each hand, palms facing toward thighs.

Action

Slowly pull the dumbbells up along the front of your body for two counts until shoulder height, so that it looks like you are making a victory shape.
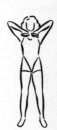
* Elbows high
* Wrists straight
* Shoulders relaxed

ANTERIOR DELTOID: FRONT SHOULDER

This exercise can be carried out in sitting or standing position. With correct posture, extend your arms down in front of you with dumbbells in each hand, palms facing the thighs. Make sure your back is straight. Raise both arms or one at a time.

Action

Raise your arm slowly in front of you for two counts until shoulder height and then lower two counts.
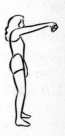
* Make sure you don't go beyond shoulder level
* Make your actions slow, smooth and controlled

LATERAL RAISES: DELTOID (SHOULDERS)

These very important muscles give you that wonderful 'shoulder pad' look – essential for upper body shaping. These exercises can be carried out in standing or sitting position. With correct posture, hold a dumbbell in each hand with the palms facing inwards. Keep the arms straight but not locked.

Action

Raise the dumbbells slowly sideways to shoulder level for two counts and gently lower two counts.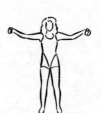

* Do not swing the weights
* Do not take above shoulder level
* Elbows should be higher than wrist

PULL OVERS: PECTORALS AND LATISSIMUS DORSI (CHEST AND BACK)

Ideally this exercise needs some form of a bench. However, if you don't have one, use your bed, lying with your head at the end.

Lie on your back, knees bent, feet flat. Elbows bent by your side and your dumbbell in both hands in front of your abdomen.

Action

Raise your hands to make a semi-circle so that your weight drops comfortably behind your head. Now slowly lift the weight back in a semi-circle to starting position.

* Keep your abdomen tight so that your lower back is in a stable position
* Make sure you don't hunch your shoulders as you lift your arms over your head

REMEMBER TO STRETCH YOUR UPPER BACK (PAGE 87), SHOULDERS (PAGE 88), CHEST (PAGE 87) AND BACK (PAGE 88).

THE A-TYPE

The A-type needs to do aerobic work to keep her ideal body weight and to prevent unwanted fat accumulating around her middle and upper body: one of the prime causes of back ache, round shoulders and poor posture. We are also now aware that abdominal fat not only compromises posture but is a health risk later in life.

Cardiovascular activity is of prime importance for this body type. Any cardiovascular activity is suitable. If you are a sporty A-type, why not take up a sport such as hockey or netball, or even running? If you don't want to become over-muscular or powerful-looking, avoid high-resistance activities that build up the upper body, such as lifting heavy weights. Do the general exercises to develop and maintain good tone, but also do the following core exercises to ensure good posture and to promote that naturally good shape you have. Do 2 sets of each exercise, with a suitable weight that will allow you to do around 15 repetitions.

SEATED ROW: RHOMBOIDS AND POSTERIOR DELTOID

Try this exercise without weights first to ensure correct posture and good technique. Then move on to using weights. Sit on the second step of your stairs or on a step with your feet flat on the floor and your knees bent. Rest your chest on your thighs.

Action
Holding your weights in each hand, with hands by your ankles, pull your elbows towards you and squeeze your shoulder blades together.

* Make sure you keep your back straight
* Lead with the elbows

PEC DEC: PECTORALS

This exercise is good for posture and works the chest muscles to ensure good musculature to support the bust. Lie on your back with knees bent and feet flat on the floor. Place your arms on the floor beside you with elbows bent in line with the shoulders.

Action

Bring both arms in front of the chest so that you press the forearms and hands tightly together for two counts, and then bring the arms slowly back to the side.
* Keep the forearm and wrist on the floor at starting position
* Relax shoulders

REVERSE CURLS: ABDOMINALS

The target area for this body type is the abdominals. Not only will abdominal exercise give you a flatter shape, it contributes enormously to good posture by supporting the lower back. The following exercise works the lower part of the abdominals and can be added to the abdominal exercises in the posture and general exercise chapters. Build up to 20 reps, then rest and repeat.

Lie on your back with knees bent, feet flat on the floor. Now bring your knees over your abdominals and in line with your tummy button. Relax your arms by your sides in a comfortable position.

Action

Use your abdominals to tilt your pelvis up towards the ceiling for two counts, then gently release two counts, holding

abdominals in all the time.
* Do not strain the upper body
* Make sure the knees stay over the tummy button
* Do not swing or rock your legs
* Ensure that your back remains on the floor

TRICEPS: BACK OF THE ARM

Another target area for the A-type is the back of the upper arm. Excess weight can make the back of the upper arm look flabby, especially as you get older. Along with aerobic exercise to lose weight, the following exercise will give those muscles at the back of the upper arm the lift they need.

Sitting on the floor with knees bent, place your hands behind you with fingers facing forward. Make sure elbows face away from you. Take your body weight on to your arms.

Action
Bend the elbows, taking your body weight on to the arms. Now straighten the arms without locking the elbows and repeat.
* Don't hunch your shoulders
* Keep your back straight
** Advanced variation: lift your bottom off the floor

REMEMBER TO STRETCH YOUR UPPER BACK (PAGE 87), CHEST (PAGE 87), ABDOMINALS (PAGE 89) AND TRICEPS (PAGE 90).

THE T-TYPE

This is the body type that can build muscle without worrying about looking bulky. For a curvier shape, the T-type needs to focus on toning and increasing muscle. Although this is the dominant part of her exercise programme, she also needs to do cardiovascular work for heart and lung fitness and to maintain that fast metabolism with age: aerobic activity three times a week is good.

Start with aerobic work at a moderate intensity and build a good base level of fitness. Once you have achieved this, build on your cardiovascular fitness and increase your muscle mass by intensifying your workout and choosing activities which incorporate resistance, such as interval training, circuit training, swimming, rowing, stationary cycling or stepping at a higher resistance. Because of the higher intensity and resistance you may not be able to sustain these activities long unless you have built up a good base level of fitness.

For shaping, slowly build up strength by following the core exercises for your type. Start by working without weights and putting mind to muscle to learn good form, and then start to add resistance by using light weights, progressing gradually to heavier weights with fewer repetitions.

Do the general exercises three times a week along with the core exercises, beginning with one exercise per body part then building on that. Use weights or resistance that will allow you to complete 10 to 12 repetitions. The exercises in the core section are especially designed to shape the legs and to maintain and develop good posture.

DECLINE PRESS-UP: UPPER PART OF CHEST AND FRONT SHOULDER

This exercise is a variation on the box press-up (page 82) but concentrates on the upper chest and front shoulder as well as the triceps so that the shoulders become stronger and more shapely. Build up your base level of fitness on the box press-up before attempting this one.

Use the first step of your stairs (you could use a low sofa or bed as an alternative). Kneel with knees on the stair and hands shoulder width apart on the floor (your bottom will be higher than your shoulders).

Action

Lean forward so that your body weight is over your arms. Pull abdominals in so that your back is flat. Bend your arms for two counts to bring the front of your shoulders to the floor, and gently press back up again for two counts.

* Do not lock your arms as you come up
* Relax your shoulders
* If there is too much stress on the wrist,
  try turning your fingers out slightly

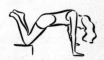

CALF SHAPER

The muscles of the lower leg are used in everyday activities and the following exercise gives them strength and shape.

Stand by a support with feet slightly apart, knees straight but not locked and abdominals in.

Action

Simply raise your heels off the ground for two counts and slowly lower two counts.
* Focus on the big and the middle toes, not the outside of the foot
* Keep your legs straight not bent
** Variation: advanced. Wrap your left foot round your right ankle. Keeping the right leg straight, raise the right heel off the ground for two counts.

FORWARD LUNGE: QUADRICEPS, HAMSTRING, GLUTEALS

This exercise focuses on the muscles of the front thigh, back thigh and bottom. Start the exercise without holding a weight to begin with for correct technique. When you can do at least 15 reps with ease, start to progress by increasing the resistance with dumbbells.

Stand with feet together in correct posture.

Action

Take one step forward and bend both knees so that you are making a right angle. Now push yourself up through your front leg to standing position.

* Hold abdominals in
* Keep back flat
* Make sure the front knee is in line with the toes
* Do not allow the knee to go over the toes
* You should not feel strain on the knees
* Make sure the back heel comes off the ground

REVERSE FLY: RHOMBOIDS AND POSTERIOR DELTOID

Good posture means strong balanced chest and back muscles. The best way to improve posture is to counteract all tendencies to hunch by exercising the back muscles. This simple exercise focuses on the rhomboids and posterior deltoid. As you perform the move, keep a balance between left and right sides. (Most people are one-side dominant.)

Lie face down with your legs straight and arms out to sides at shoulder level. Keeping your arms flat to the floor, bend your elbows so your upper and lower arms are at right angles and hands are roughly level with your head.

Action

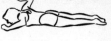

Leading with the elbow, lift your arms and squeeze the shoulder blades together two counts and release two counts.

* Keep hips and feet to the floor
* Don't jerk as you lift
* Keep chin tucked in and head in line with your spine

REMEMBER TO STRETCH YOUR CHEST (PAGE 87), CALVES (PAGE 78), FRONT THIGH (PAGE 79) AND BACK THIGH (PAGE 78).

THE P-TYPE

Endurance work is the vital exercise prescription for the P-type. The P-type needs to burn calories to get rid of the excess body fat which tends to accumulate all over. Choose aerobic activities at low to moderate intensity for long duration such as fast walking, aerobics, cycling (with low resistance). Dancing and endurance-based circuit training are also good. Avoid muscle bulking by cutting out high-resistance aerobic work on a high setting on a stationary bike or stepping machine. Also avoid lifting heavy weights.

This body type needs to work upper and lower body evenly, sticking to light weights that allow 15 to 20 reps. Do all the general exercises and the following core exercises. The exercises that I have chosen are to maintain and develop good posture, and for leaner, stronger, more shapely legs.

PLIÉ SQUAT: THIGHS AND BOTTOM

The plié squat is a squat with a difference in that it works front thigh, back thigh and the gluteal muscles. Take your legs wider than shoulder-width apart, and turn your toes out at ten to and ten past the hour.

Action
Bend your knees out in line with your toes and slowly push through your heels to straighten up again.

* Pull your abdominals in
* You should not feel strain on your knee
* Don't arch your back
* Keep your head up at all times

CHEST FLY: PECTORALS

This exercise works to combat a top-heavy posture by strengthening and supporting the muscles around the chest, giving the bust a more lifted appearance. Ideally you need a bench or step or equivalent surface. Alternatively, lie on the floor, although this will impede range of movement.

Lie on your back with knees bent, feet flat on the floor. With dumbbells in each hand, extend your arms over your head so they are above the shoulders. Make sure the wrists are facing each other.

Action
Bend elbows slightly. Make a semi-circle by taking the arms out to the side in line with the chest.

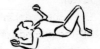

* Practice this exercise without weights
  initially to ensure good technique

BACK SQUEEZE: RHOMBOID TRAPEZIUS

Good posture means strong, balanced muscles. You can do a lot to create this balance by ensuring you include opposite muscle groups in your exercise programme. Opposite to the chest muscles (exercised in the chest fly) are the muscles in the back.

Sit upright on a chair, fairly close to the edge, with feet together and good posture. Reach forward and upwards with arms out at shoulder level.

Action

Pull your arms towards you in a diagonal line and squeeze your shoulder blades together as you do so.
* Try to relax shoulders, head and neck
* Lead with elbows
* Make sure the body remains upright throughout

ABDOMINALS

As well as aerobic exercise you need abdominal exercise to keep the body in good alignment. This exercise isolates the abdominal muscles to give them an intense workout.

Lie on your back with your feet up against a wall. The knees should be just be over your tummy and in line with your hips to make a right angle. Place both hands at the side of your head for support. Pull your abdominals in.

Action

Use your abdominals to lift your shoulders off the ground for two counts. Gently lower. Make sure you don't pull on your head. Keep the abdominals in tight.

REMEMBER TO STRETCH YOUR FRONT THIGH (PAGE 79), BACK THIGH (PAGE 78), CHEST (PAGE 87), UPPER BACK (PAGE 87) AND ABDOMINALS (PAGE 89).

CHAPTER TEN

Developing a
Personal Programme

E ach body type needs to perform their exercises within a realistic framework or timetable to ensure a balanced and consistent programme. For instance, if G-, A- and P-types need to lose weight, they will have to do aerobic exercise, which may be quite time-consuming. If you were to do your toning on the same day as your aerobic work, you might be spending too much time exercising, which could lead to boredom and dropout.

The following programmes offer variety for each body type, combining all that you have learnt so far to enable you to complete exercise sessions successfully and in a balanced way. The programmes, which are made up of four sessions spread over a week with rest days between, show how to progress from being a complete beginner to someone with a base level of fitness. Once this base level of fitness has been achieved, you are then shown how to progress to body-shaping appropriate for you, and finally how to maintain that perfect shape.

The programmes are guidelines. While it is important to be committed to achieving your goals, it is also essential to do what you realistically can in terms of time and effort. You may not be able to do as much as is recommended. If you can't, that's fine. Don't give up, just modify the programmes to your needs, trying to be consistent with what you can do. It may take a little longer but you will still get there.

You may have to combine sessions, or make certain you exercise core body parts on certain days. That's fine too, as long as you manage to achieve balance by working opposite muscle groups, and as long as you don't exercise the same muscle two days running. A day's rest is needed before exercising the same muscle group.

> *While it is important to be committed to achieving your goals, it is also essential to do what you realistically can in terms of time and effort*

You do not have to include all your core exercises in your programme at once. Indeed, it may be better not to. For instance, if a G-type was to do all the shoulder exercises at once, she may end up with a neck ache and overworked shoulder muscles. Start off by exercising one body part at a time and then gradually build the core exercises into your general exercise programme. Make sure you build up to no more than two to three exercises per body part.

For weight loss you need ideally to work aerobically during three to five sessions per week. If time or inclination allows, then five sessions; otherwise, three or four. You can also help burn calories by making your lifestyle more active: for example, walk instead of drive, take the stairs instead of the lift. Remember, the more you move the more calories you burn.

You may find some exercises too easy. For the complete beginner, in the exercises you find really easy, use light weights (such as small bottles of water or cans of baked beans), and put your mind into your muscles to create as much tension and resistance as possible. For those who are exercising at a more general level and are using dumbbells, increase the resistance in easier exercises by using heavier weights. Remember to work on the principle of overload. At the end of each exercise you should feel your muscles really working. If you don't, you need to progress. Monitor your progression by using your own awareness, as well as the talk test and the heart-rate monitoring described on page 36. (The only person you can cheat is yourself!)

If you find some of the exercises difficult, focus on gradual building. If you can only do a few of an exercise, that's fine. You will find that a week later you will

> *The key to success is to work at your own pace*

be able to do a few more. The key to success is to work at your own pace, and you will find that you succeed!

G-TYPE PERSONAL PROGRAMME

This programme concentrates on building up the G-type's strength and endurance to achieve a base level of fitness. From here you can advance towards the goal of a streamlined lower body and a more balanced upper body. The aerobic sessions are for heart and lung fitness and to burn calories to make you a slimmer G-type. The G-type shouldn't do too much too soon, so the aerobic sessions are built gradually into the programme in order to challenge but still to keep progression comfortable. At this point the G-type needs to be working at about 55 to 60 per cent of maximum heart rate.

The strength section starts with one set and progresses to two at week 5. I have split the workout here into upper body work one session and lower the next. This is time management, and can mean the difference between success and dropout.

The programme is spread over four days out of seven. It is OK to do aerobic work two days in a row, but not strength exercises with the same muscle groups. Aim for at least one day's rest after each day of exercise.

A	Aerobics (minutes)
C	Conditioning (sets x reps)
UB	Upper body
LB	Lower body
FB	Full body

WEEK	DAY 1	DAY 2	DAY 3	DAY 4
1	A 10	C 1x10	REST	A 10 & C 1x10
2	A 12	C 1x12	REST	A 12 & C 1x12
3	A 12/15	A 12–15 & C 1x12–15	REST	A 12–15 & C 1x12–15
4	A 15	A 15 & C 1x15	REST	A 15 & C 1x15
5	A 17 & C 2x10 UB	A 17 & C 2x10 LB	REST	A 17 & C 2x10 FB
6	A 20 & C 2x10 UB	A 20 & C 2x10 LB	REST	A 20 & C 2x10 FB
7	A 20 & C 2x12 UB	A 20 & C 2x12 LB	A 20 & C 2x12 UB	A 20 & C 2x12 LB
8	A 20 & C 2x12 UB	A 20 & C 2x12 LB	A 20 & C 2x12 UB	A 20 & C 2x12 LB
9	A 20 & C 2x12–15 UB	A 20 & C 2x12–15 UB	A 20 & C 2x12–15 UB	A 20 & C 2x12–15 LB
10	A 20 & C 2x15 UB	A 20 & C 2x15 LB	A 20 & C 2x15 UB	A 20 & C 2x15 LB

PROGRESSION

When the G-type has completed her ten-week programme and reached a base level of fitness, she can progress. The advantage for all beginners to exercise is that good fitness results are generally seen within the first three months of exercising. Thereafter, the body tends to plateau and needs to be challenged in some way. For the G-type, this is the ideal opportunity to focus on sculpting the upper body for a more curvy but balanced look.

After the ten-week programme the G-type needs to increase the weight load to work the upper body for 10 to 12 repetitions, while increasing the duration of exercise to the lower body to 15 to 20 repetitions. When this becomes easy, start a third set of reps or add light resistance. It is important not to use heavy weights for the lower body as this will result in a bulky look, especially if you have a lot of weight to lose. It is also important to ensure you do not overload the shoulders when initially working with a heavier weight. Again, build those core exercises progressively into the programme.

The G-type needs to progress aerobically to burn optimum calories – so increase the duration of your activities to 30 or even 40 minutes, or increase the intensity of your workout.

MAINTENANCE

When the G-type reaches her goal she will need to maintain her shape and her fitness levels. Maintenance requires less frequency and duration of exercise but it is really important to keep up the intensity in order to achieve the necessary over-load. So focus on aerobic exercise three times a week, and one or two toning sessions per week, with 10 to 12 reps for the upper body and 15 to 20 reps for the lower body.

A-TYPE PERSONAL PROGRAMME

If the A-type needs to lose weight she needs to do between three and five aerobic sessions per week. She also needs to work her abdominals for posture and good shape. In this pro-gramme you do abdominal work on each one of the sessions. On the aerobic days she also does the curl and oblique exer-cises from the general chapter and the reverse curl from the core exercises. On the toning days she works on the trans-verse abdominal exercises in the posture section. Build up to 25 reps of each abdominal exercise, paying attention to tech-nique and ensuring that your back is not arched.

Build the core exercises into the general exercises and

when you get to week 5, split the sessions so that on one day you are working your back, biceps and shoulders and on another you are working chest, triceps and legs. Remember abdominals both days.

A	Aerobics (minutes)
C	Conditioning (sets x reps)
BBS	Back, biceps, shoulders
CTL	Chest, triceps, legs
Abs	Abdominals
FB	Full body

WEEKS	DAY 1	DAY 2	DAY 3	DAY 4
1	A 10 & C 1x10 Abs	REST	A 10 & C 1x10 Abs	REST
2	A 12 & C 1x12 Abs	REST	A 12 & C 1x12 Abs	REST
3	A 12–15 & C 1x12 Abs	REST	A 12–15 & C 1x12 Abs	A12–15
4	A 15 & C 1x15 Abs	REST	A 15 & C 1x15 Abs	A15
5	A 17 & C 2x10 FB	REST	A 17 & C 2x10 CTL Abs	A 17 & C 2x10 BBS Abs
6	A 20 & C 2x10 FB	REST	A 20 & C 2x10 CTL Abs	A 20 & C 2x10 BBS Abs
7	A 20 & C 2x12 CTL Abs	A 20 & C 2x12 BBS Abs	A 20 & C 2x12 CTL Abs	A 20 & C 2x12 BBS Abs
8	A 20 & C 2x12 CTL Abs	A 20 & C 2x12 BBS Abs	A 20 & C 2x12 CTL Abs	A 20 & C 2x12 BBS Abs
9	A 20 & C 2x12–15 CTL Abs	A 20 & C 2x12–15 BBS Abs	A 20 & C 2x12–15 CTL Abs	A 20 & C 2x12–15 BBS Abs
10	A 20 & C 2x15 CTL Abs	A 20 & C 2x15 BBS Abs	A 20 & C 2x15 CTL Abs	A 20 & C 2x15 BBS Abs

PROGRESSION

On finishing the ten-week programme, the A-type needs to stick to a strength and endurance programme unless she has a specific goal to build muscles. Keep working to 15 reps, increasing to a third set when two sets are easy. You can also add more resistance in the form of hand weights or light ankle weights. For a more muscular look you should work with a heavier weight at 10 to 12 repetitions.

The A-type also needs to progress aerobically, and to do this you can increase either duration or intensity. Think about adding variations to the programme for motivation – cross training, for example: combining different activities into a session or changing from one to another, such as from walking to a gentle jog or from cycling to swimming. Add all the core exercises to the general programme and keep up the abdominal work.

MAINTENANCE

The A-type needs to do three aerobic sessions of 20 or 30 minutes per week, working on increasing the intensity. Aim to work at 70 per cent maximum heart rate. She also needs to do one or two toning sessions per week, working with weights that will allow her to do 15 reps.

T-TYPE PERSONAL PROGRAMME

The T-type should aim to do no more than three full-body toning sessions per week, gradually incorporating core exercises into the general ones. You also need to do aerobic exercise for heart and lung fitness, but no more than three aerobic sessions per week, as the aim is not to lose weight.

The T-type needs to work at a moderate intensity that will allow her to be just out of breath: 50 to 60 per cent of maximum heart rate. If you are an underweight T-type, you need to consume extra calories to make up for the ones you have lost: eat an extra 500 calories after aerobic exercise.

I have devised a programme of two full-body toning sessions a week and three aerobic sessions for heart and lung fitness. When the T-type introduces weights into her programme, she needs to choose a weight that it not so heavy it might cause strain and injury, but not so light that it offers little resistance. Remember not to work the same body parts two days running.

A	Aerobics (minutes)
C	Conditioning (sets x reps)
UB	Upper body
LB	Lower body
FB	Full body

WEEKS	DAY 1	DAY 2	DAY 3	DAY 4
1	C 1x10	A 10	C 1x10	REST
2	C 1x12	A 12	A 12 & C 1x12	REST
3	A 12–15 & C 1x12–15	A 12–15	A 12–15 & C 1x12–15	REST
4	A 15 & C 1x15	A 15	A 15 & C 1x15	REST
5	A 17 & C 2x10 UB	A 17 & C 2x10 LB	A 17	C 2x10 FB
6	A 20 & C 2x10 UB	A 20 & C 2x10 LB	A 20	C 2x10 FB
7	A 20 & C 2x12 UB	A 20 & C 2x12 LB	A 20	C 2x12 FB
8	A 20 & C 2x12 UB	A 20 & C 2x12 LB	A 20	C 2x12 FB
9	A 20 & C 2x12–15 UB	A 20 & C 2x12–15 LB	A 20	C 2x12–15 FB
10	A 20 & C 2x15 UB	A 20 & C 2x15 LB	A 20	C 2x 15 FB

PROGRESSION

Once the T-type has progressed to ten weeks and built a base level of fitness, she can focus on a strength-training programme that will allow her to build muscles without bulking.

Work with weights that allow 10 to 12 reps for all-over body sculpting. I strongly recommend that, if this is not possible at home, you join a gym that has progressive-resistance machines and free weights. For building muscle, you may want to build more than one exercise per body part into your programme. When I was working to build, I incorporated two and progressed to three exercises per body part.

The T-type also needs to progress aerobically. Do this by increasing the intensity of the workout to 70 per cent maximum heart rate. If short on time, add resistance to the aerobic programme with activities such as circuit training or cross training. Rowing, stair master or stationary cycling with added resistance would all be ideal.

Remember to add an extra 500 calories to your diet when working out aerobically so as not to lose weight.

MAINTENANCE

To maintain your new curvy shape, do one or two toning sessions per week, remembering to keep up the intensity so that the last few repetitions really count. Maintain aerobic fitness with three cardiovascular sessions per week.

P-TYPE PERSONAL PROGRAMME

The P-type needs to have a predominately endurance programme. She needs to work out aerobically between three and five times per week for weight loss.

This programme builds up to four aerobic sessions per week, working at 50 to 60 maximum heart rate. The strength programme is twice a week but again is split into front-of-body workouts (chest, biceps, abdominals) and back-of-body workouts (shoulders, back, triceps) on alternate days. Do abdominal work in all sessions. When it comes to the legs, do squats one day and then inner and outer thigh the next, or do them both on the same day.

It is entirely up to you to build these exercises into your lifestyle to make your goals achievable. Remember to build core exercises into the general exercise session for shape, strength and posture, and train, don't strain! Don't drive your body too hard. Overtraining leads to injuries to muscles and joints, and can also cause fatigue, insomnia and loss of appetite. Make sure you tailor your fitness programme to your needs, and think long term rather than short. Work at an intensity that is comfortable: 55 to 70 per cent of maximum heart rate.

A	Aerobics (minutes)
C	Conditioning (sets x reps)
F	Front body
B	Back body

WEEKS	DAY 1	DAY 2	DAY 3	DAY 4
1	A 10 & C 1x10	REST	A 10 & C 1x10	REST
2	A 12 & C 1x12	REST	A 12 & C 1x12	REST
3	A 12–15 & C 1x12–15	REST	A 12–15 & C 1x12–15	A 12–15
4	A 15 & C 1x15	REST	A 15 & C 1x15	A 15
5	A 17	C 2x10	A 17 & C 2x10 F	A 17 & C 2x10 B

6	A 20	C 2x10	A 20 & C 2x10 F	A 20 & C 2x10 B
7	A 20 & C 2x10 F	A 20 & C 2x10 B	A 20 & C 2x10 F	A 20 & C 2x10 B
8	A 20 & C 2x12 F	A 20 & C 2x12 B	A 20 & C 2x12 F	A 20 & C 2x12 B
9	A 20 & C 2x12–15 F	A 20 & C 2x12–15 B	A 20 & C 2x12–15 F	A 20 & C 2x12–15 B
10	A 20 & C 2x15 F	A 20 & C 2x15 B	A 20 & C 2x15 F	A 20 & C 2x15 B

PROGRESSION

When the P-type can do more than 20 minutes of aerobic activity with ease, progress slowly and gradually up to 30 minutes and even 40 to burn more calories, working at 50 to 70 per cent maximum heart rate. Look at varying your routine so that you remain motivated and do not plateau. Instead of increasing resistance, progress from 15 repetitions to 20 repetitions, moving from one body part to another. When you can complete two sets of 20 reps, move to three sets.

MAINTENANCE

For maintenance the P-type needs to make a concerted lifestyle habit of three aerobic sessions per week and one to two strength sessions. Remember to work at an intensity that is challenging but does not compromise good technique.

CHAPTER ELEVEN

You Are
What You Eat

I wonder how many times we have heard that we are what we eat. Well, it is true. The way we look, act and feel depends very much on our fuel source – the food we eat and drink. In the past, food advice tended to be general. We are all familiar with the guidelines: low fat, high carbohydrate, moderate amounts of protein and plenty of fruit and vegetables. While these guidelines still apply to a certain degree, it appears that there is much more to the equation.

Science now shows that our four body types have metabolisms with different dietary needs. This is an important part of the Apples and Pears fitness programme: an individual eating plan on top of a tailor-made exercise programme are together instrumental in helping each type find their perfect shape.

BODY TYPES AND METABOLISM

We all process food differently. Some people might thrive on a certain food while others respond less favourably. Some people put on weight very quickly while others can eat and eat and not pile on the pounds. Some people need more of different types of food like carbohydrate or proteins while others need less.

Each of our body types has a metabolic weakness caused by the tendency to stimulate the dominant hormonal gland, usually by eating the wrong food. This can potentially result in weight gain or health problems. To achieve metabolic balance in the body, you need to reduce the foods that stimulate your dominant hormonal gland to become overactive, and increase the foods that support and strengthen the less active glands.

Each of our body types also has a 'best' time of the day, when the dominant gland is most active and when the main meal of the day is best digested.

WHAT IS IN FOOD

Food provides energy and essential nutrients to keep you going and for growth and renewal of the body tissues. It can play an important part in health, either contributing to or reducing the risk of heart disease, blood pressure, cancer and obesity. In exercise, energy is needed as fuel for your muscles. Proper nutrition is an important part of an exercise programme, and bad eating habits can prevent you from reaching your full potential. The more finely tuned and specific to your body type your nutritional programme is, the more likely you are to have increased energy, better performance in exercise, improved health, and of course success in achieving your ideal body weight.

The body requires different types of food to supply the tissues with nutrients for energy. Food is made up of proteins, fats and carbohydrates, and each of these contains calories and can be used by the body in different ways. These calories can be used for heat, for movement, to build and to be stored as fat. We also use water, fibre, vitamins and minerals.

The table shows the energy per gram of each of the main nutrients. It shows how fat is denser in calories than carbohydrate and protein.

ENERGY PER GRAM

1 gram carbohydrate	4 calories
1 gram fat	9 calories
1 gram protein	4 calories

CARBOHYDRATES

Carbohydrate comes in two forms, simple sugars and complex carbohydrates.

Simple sugars provide energy but no other nutrients and are absorbed quickly into the bloodstream. When we take in this form of energy, the body must work to keep its level of blood sugar within normal limits. It can easily end up with more energy than it can use immediately and it will store the excess as fat. There is also the danger of tooth decay. Simple sugars, often combined with fats, come in the form of cakes, biscuits, desserts, sweetened drinks and chocolate bars.

SIMPLE SUGARS

sugar, syrup, glucose, fructose, milk, honey, jam, sweets, sugar-coating, such as on cereal

Complex carbohydrates, formerly known as starch, come in the form of bread, pasta, rice, potatoes, vegetables and some fruits. This form of carbohydrate takes longer to break down in the digestive system and provides a slower release of energy over a longer period of time – much more beneficial than simple sugars.

Complex carbohydrates are fuel for the muscles and the major energy source of the body. When broken down they are stored in the muscles and liver as glycogen, to be used as energy. If you are a regular exerciser and eat a diet that is low in carbohydrates, the energy in your muscles can become reduced. This will result in poor performance and also contribute to feelings of tiredness and fatigue.

EXAMPLES OF COMPLEX CARBOHYDRATES

rice, potatoes, bread, pasta, bananas, porridge, apples, wholegrain products, corn

QUESTION: Should I have soft drinks or sweets or sugar before exercise?

The body responds to simple sugars entering the bloodstream by increasing insulin levels. This can cause blood sugar levels to drop, and result in the exerciser feeling tired and weak. To boost energy levels eat complex carbohydrates instead, two to three hours before exercise: they add sugars more slowly and sustainably to the bloodstream.

PROTEIN

Next to water, protein is the largest component of the body. Present in every cell, including the skin, nails, bones, cartilage and of course the muscles, protein plays a fundamental part in growth and repair of the body's tissues. During digestion, protein food is broken down into amino acids, which are released into the bloodstream to be used within the body.

A common misunderstanding is that it is important to eat large amounts of protein. Many active people eat much more than they need in the hope of building stronger and bigger muscles. However, excess protein eaten isn't stored by the body as protein. It is either stored as fat or used for energy, and protein is an inefficient source of energy. Carbohydrate is the better source.

Eating too much protein can cause weight gain and dehydration. Excessive protein may also place a heavy burden on the liver and kidneys.

PROTEIN

Protein comes in the form of:

meat, fish, eggs, cheese (also high in fat), soya beans, peanuts, poultry, lentils, kidney beans

FATS

The final source of calories in your diet is fat. Believe it or not, some fat in the diet is essential. Fat in the body

> *Believe it or not, some fat in the diet is essential*

is vital for the protection of our internal organs and also acts as a carrier for fat-soluble vitamins such as A and E, as well as vitamins D and K. We need a small amount of fat – in the diet and on our body – for good health. However, we tend to consume more than we need. The World Health Organisation recommends that no more than 30 per cent of our diet is made up of fat. Research suggests that on average we consume nearer 40 per cent.

Fat is loaded with calories. It is often 'hidden' in processed and manufactured foods to give them a palatable texture. We consume lots of it without even noticing.

Excess fat in the diet increases the risk of high blood pressure, diabetes, heart disease and obesity.

Saturated and unsaturated fats

Fats can be divided into two groups: saturated and unsaturated. Saturated fats are drawn mainly from animal sources, for example, butter and cream. The fat on meat is saturated. Concentrated saturated fat is solid at room temperature. A little saturated fat in the diet does no harm, but when used excessively can lead to obesity.

Unsaturated fats are further divided into two groups: monounsaturated and polyunsaturated. These are the preferred fats. They offer positive health benefits and need to be included in your diet. Unsaturated fats are mostly derived from plant sources: olive oil and most vegetable oils, for example. They are liquid at room temperature. The oil from oily fish such as mackerel is also a beneficial, unsaturated form of fat.

EXAMPLES OF HIGH-FAT FOODS

butter, lard, cream, fatty meat, suet, oils, dressings, peanuts, oily fish, cheese

WATER

Eating a diet high in both fruit and vegetables cleanses your body as well as supplying it with nutrients and fibre

We can survive without food for much longer than we can survive without water. Sixty per cent of our body is made up of water. It provides the fluid that is vital to the efficient functioning of the body: both intracellular (inside the cells), and extracellular (outside the cells), such as blood plasma and saliva. Water is also found in food, indeed about 90 per cent of most fruit and vegetables is water. Eating a diet high in both fruit and vegetables cleanses your body as well as supplying it with nutrients and fibre.

QUESTION: Should I drink water before exercise?

Fluids play a very important part in your training programme. When you perspire you lose fluids, which can lead to dehydration and impair your performance. You can tell if you are drinking enough water by the colour of your urine. It should be almost colourless except for first thing in the morning. It is recommended you regularly drink around 6 to 8 glasses of water a day, as well as before, during and after exercise.

FIBRE

Fibre is an essential part of a healthy-eating programme, playing a crucial role in the digestion and absorption of food. It is found in plant foods such as grains, fruit, vegetables, seeds and nuts, with the greatest concentrations found in the skins and outer coating. People who have plenty of fibre in their diet generally have a low incidence of bowel cancer, diabetes, gallstones, heart disease, obesity and constipation.

There are two types of fibre: soluble and insoluble. Soluble fibre dissolves easily in water and is partly broken down during digestion. It helps to control the uptake of sugar by the blood and to reduce cholesterol levels and high blood pressure. Insoluble fibre helps to push food through the digestive system and is instrumental in preventing conditions such constipation and diseases of the bowel.

To increase your fibre intake:
* Eat more fruit and vegetable   * Choose whole-grain products
* Increase complex carbohydrates

WHAT TO EAT

The general view is that our diet today contains more protein than is needed, not enough of the right type of carbohydrates, not enough fibre and fluids, and too much of the wrong type of fat. There are variations for each body type, but essentially any healthy-eating plan works along the same basic principles:
* Eat fewer high-fat protein foods like cheese, full-fat milk, fatty cuts of red meat
* Instead eat low-fat protein foods, such as fish, poultry and pulses
* Drink plenty of water

* Eat plenty of fresh fruit and vegetables
* Eat complex carbohydrates, such as rice, pasta and bread
* Cut out simple sugars like cakes and biscuits

BODY TYPES AND DIET

Each of our four body types has a dominant gland, which is affected by particular foods. When overstimulated, the gland produces more of its particular hormones. Over a period of time this overstimulation weakens the dominant gland, which results in health problems and weight gain. By eliminating or reducing these foods you can achieve a balance in your body, which leads to good health and a perfect shape.

DIET FOR THE G-TYPE

When a G-type eats spicy foods, she is increasing the stimulation to the gonadal area by enlarging the blood vessels there. The G-type also gets cravings for creamy fatty foods, which again has the effect of stimulating the gonads. The key to healthy eating for the G-type is to decrease stimulation to the gonads by eliminating creamy fatty foods and spices from the diet. You need a diet that is high in whole grains with moderate amounts of protein, and high in fruit and vegetables. Fruit and vegetables stimulate the thyroid, which boosts the metabolism; excellent for the G-type.

FOODS TO EAT

CARBOHYDRATES Whole grains and wholegrain products, such as brown rice, rye, oats, millet, barley, corn, whole wheat, spelt (an old variety of wheat), buckwheat; wholegrain pasta and bread; potatoes
PROTEINS Free-range poultry and eggs; fish (fresh and canned),

particularly oily fish such as herring, mackerel, sardines, salmon, tuna; lean cuts of red meat with visible fat removed before cooking
DAIRY PRODUCTS Low-fat milk, low-fat cheese, soya products, natural yoghurt, goat's or sheep's milk and yoghurt
FRUIT AND VEGETABLES All fresh and dried fruits; salad vegetables, green vegetables and root vegetables; canned fruit in natural juice or water; herbs such as dill, parsley, basil, tarragon and thyme
DRINKS Boiled water with a squeeze of lemon or lime juice to start the day; 6 to 8 glasses of filtered or mineral water throughout the day; herbal tea; juices (fruit)

FOODS TO AVOID

Refined, bleached, white-flour products such as white bread, packaged cakes and biscuits
Sugar and honey
Processed meats, bacon, sausages, commercially raised poultry and eggs, and organ meats
Full-fat milk, butter, cream, ice cream, chocolate, coconut cream, all saturated fats and oils
Deep-fried foods
Carbonated soft drinks, chocolate and malted drinks

WHEN TO EAT

For G-types it is important to start the day with a light breakfast because your metabolism handles food better later in the day. Breakfast should be a fruit and grain meal: fresh fruit, or soaked dried fruit, yoghurt, wholegrain bread or crispbread. Even though breakfast is a light meal, it is nonetheless important to have it as blood sugar levels will be low without it.

Lunch should also be light and should consist of plenty of

grains, vegetables, salad and a small amount of protein.

The evening meal is the most substantial one for the G-type because this is when your metabolism is most active. Again, lots of grains, vegetables, poultry or fish or cheese, and fruit. Try to eat early in the evening.

Snack attack

The G-type's first danger period is mid-morning when you are likely to want a quick fix of sugar. Late at night is also a danger period. Try to stick to raw fruit and vegetables.

DIET FOR THE A-TYPE

A good, healthy-eating plan for the A-type would be a diet high in complex carbohydrates, fruits and vegetables. The aim is to lower the stimulation to the adrenals and boost the activity of the pituitary and thyroid glands. To do this you need to cut out salty foods and reduce red meats, which stimulate your adrenals, and increase stimulation to the thyroid and pituitary with complex carbohydrates and light, low-fat dairy products. A vegetarian diet with grains, cereals, plenty of fruit and vegetables suits the metabolism of the A-type.

FOODS TO EAT

CARBOHYDRATES Whole grains and wholegrain products, such as brown rice, rye, oats, millet, barley, corn, whole wheat, spelt (an old variety of wheat), buckwheat; wholegrain pasta and bread; potatoes
PROTEINS Free-range poultry and eggs; fish (fresh and canned), particularly oily fish such as herring, mackerel, sardines, salmon, tuna; all types of beans, lentils, peas and tofu; unsalted nuts and seeds
DAIRY PRODUCTS Low-fat milk, low-fat cheese, soya products, natural yoghurt, goat's or sheep's milk and yoghurt

FRUIT AND VEGETABLES All fruits; salad vegetables; green vegetables and root vegetables; tomatoes
FATS Olive, corn and linseed oil in small amounts
DRINKS Boiled water with a squeeze of lemon or lime juice to start the day; 6 to 8 glasses of filtered or mineral water throughout the day; herbal tea; fruit juices

FOODS TO AVOID

Refined, bleached, white-flour products such as white bread, packaged cakes and biscuits

Too much sugar and honey

Excessive red meats, organ meat, processed meats, bacon, sausage, fried meats

Salt and salty foods

All full-fat dairy products, including chocolate, cream, cheese, butter and ice cream

Artificial additives, such as preservatives, and artificial sweeteners

WHEN TO EAT

Avoid eating a huge breakfast in the morning. Eat fruit, cereal or wholegrain toast and low-fat dairy products.

Lunch is a predominately light, vegetable, grain, salad meal with lots of salad, whole grains, a small amount of protein and lots of fresh fruits to keep the appetite under control.

Your most substantial meal is best in the evening as the adrenals are at their most active then. Eat poultry, fish, vegetables and fruit.

Snack attack

The adrenals' activity increases as the day progresses and your danger period is late afternoon when tiredness sets in. If you get a craving for something, try a yoghurt.

DIET FOR THE P-TYPE

The P-type needs an eating plan to stimulate a sluggish metabolism. Your weakness is lack of strength in the adrenals and gonads, which can be helped by avoiding thyroid stimulation, and by stimulating the adrenals and the gonads. The most stimulating adrenal foods are high-protein foods, found in lean cuts of red meat, poultry, fish and organ meat.

The metabolism of the P-type works most efficiently when all dairy products are eliminated. The pituitary is at its most active during the day so the best time to eat a substantial meal is in the morning or at lunchtime. When you wake in the morning have a large glass of water with a squeeze of lemon or lime juice to cleanse your system.

FOODS TO EAT

CARBOHYDRATES Whole grains and wholegrain products, such as brown rice, rye, oats, millet, barley, corn, whole wheat, spelt (an old variety of wheat), buckwheat; potatoes; crispbreads
PROTEIN Lean cuts of red meat, free-range poultry and eggs; fish (fresh or canned), especially oily fish such as herring, mackerel, sardines, salmon, tuna; organ meats; unsalted nuts and seeds, especially linseeds; tahini and raw nut pastes
FRUIT AND VEGETABLES All fresh and dried fruits; salad vegetables, green vegetables and root vegetables; canned fruit in natural juice or water
FATS Small amounts of olive oil and dairy-free margarine; linseed and pure rape seed (canola) oil in moderation
DRINKS Boiled water with a squeeze of lemon or lime juice to start the day; 6 to 8 glasses of filtered or mineral water throughout the day; herbal tea; drinks low in caffeine and tannic acid

FOODS TO AVOID

Refined, bleached, white-flour products such as white bread, packaged cakes and biscuits

Sugar and honey; fruit in sugar syrup, glazed fruit

Processed meats

All dairy products; substitute with rice milk or low-fat soya milk and soya products

Refined, bleached, white-flour products such as white bread, packaged cakes and biscuits

Carbonated soft drinks, malted and chocolate drinks, alcohol

High-fat foods

Salt and salty food

Artificial additives, such as preservatives and colours

WHEN TO EAT

The P-type needs to do the reverse of the G- and A-type. You need to eat a substantial breakfast, a moderate lunch and a light dinner.

A substantial protein breakfast will stimulate the adrenal gland: eat free-range eggs or fish with whole grain bread, herbal tea or water.

For lunch, try poultry, oily fish or red meat, cooked vegetables or a large green salad, with whole grains such as brown rice, bread or crispbread, and a piece of fresh fruit.

The evening meal should be light as the metabolism is sluggish then. Try a small amount of protein food, with vegetables and salad.

Snack attack

The P-type is most likely to snack late afternoon when the pituitary gland becomes less active. Now is the time to resist the craving for ice cream, yoghurt, cheese, sugary snacks. Have a raw vegetable: either carrots or celery.

DIET FOR THE T-TYPE

When the T-type eats the wrong food, the thyroid gland is overstimulated, making you feel tired, stressed, irritable and prone to mood swings. The thyroid gland is in charge of oxidation, or the burning of food in the tissues. Your metabolic rate is high and you burn calories very quickly.

The T-type needs to have three substantial meals a day with protein in every meal. The protein foods will stimulate and build up the adrenals and moderate your metabolism. Avoid quick-fix stimulants, such as coffee, chocolate or sugar, that will overstimulate your thyroid. The T-type diet should be high in protein and vegetable, with moderate amounts of carbohydrate. Morning is the best time to eat a substantial meal.

FOODS TO EAT

CARBOHYDRATES Whole grains and wholegrain products, such as brown rice, rye, oats, millet, barley, corn, whole wheat, spelt (an old variety of wheat), buckwheat; wholegrain pasta and bread; potatoes
PROTEINS Free-range poultry and eggs; fish (fresh and canned), particularly oily fish such as herring, mackerel, sardines, salmon, tuna; all types of beans, lentils, peas, beansprouts, tofu; unsalted raw nuts and seeds tahini and raw nut pastes
DAIRY PRODUCTS Most dairy products: mild cheeses, sheep's and goat's milk and yoghurt, low-salt feta cheese
FRUIT AND VEGETABLES All fresh and dried fruits, especially hard fruits; canned fruit in natural juice or water; a wide variety of fresh vegetables
DRINKS Boiled water with a squeeze of lemon or lime juice to start the day; 6 to 8 glasses of filtered or mineral water throughout the day; herbal tea

FOODS TO AVOID

Refined, bleached, white-flour products such as white bread, packaged cakes and biscuits

Sugar, honey, chocolate; fruit in sugar syrup, glazed fruit

Processed meats

Meat dripping, clarified butter and lard

Salt and salty food

Carbonated soft drinks, cola drinks containing caffeine, coffee, chocolate drinks

Foods containing artificial additives, preservatives and colours; foods containing MSG

WHEN TO EAT

Breakfast should be the most substantial meal of the day with high protein and whole grains, such as: eggs, oily fish and wholemeal bread.

Lunch should be a moderate meal of protein (meat, poultry or fish), vegetables and salad, a little cheese, fruit.

In the evening, eat a similar meal to lunch.

Snack attack

You are most likely to crave a stimulant of some sort in the late afternoon. Avoid chocolate or sweets. Have an egg to stimulate your adrenals and moderate your metabolism.

QUESTION: Is caffeine bad for you?

Different body types metabolise caffeine in a different way. T-types are better off without caffeine because it stimulates the thyroid. Other body types, however, can have small amounts of caffeine because they can benefit from the thyroid stimulation.

CHAPTER TWELVE

A Healthy Mind

Wе now know that doing the exercises and eating the foods appropriate for our body type will go a long way towards maximising our assets. Now, last but by no means least, is the final ingredient to help us on our way: a healthy mind.

Exercise brings about physiological changes which affect us mentally and psychologically, promoting a sense of wellbeing,

> Doing the exercises and eating the foods appropriate for our body type will go a long way towards maximising our assets

a release of tension and improved mental functioning. By taking a mindful approach to exercise, we can also use the conditioning of the mind to give us the discipline to exercise and to create a more effective workout.

Today science takes a holistic approach to health. Each person is seen as a whole unit, made up of interrelated parts which are physical, mental and emotional. It is now thought that physical and mental illness are related to each other, and treatment is often given both physically and psychologically to combat health problems. Exercise is prescribed to combat conditions such as depression, anxiety and stress, as well as to fight off physical conditions such as obesity, diabetes and osteoporosis.

Movement begins not in the muscles and bones but in the brain: it is our mind that makes us move in the first place.

Triggered by thoughts and feelings, the brain carries impulses through the autonomic nervous system, the system which controls the involuntary (spontaneous) actions of breathing, cardiac muscle activity and the movement of the intestines. The

Exercise is prescribed to combat conditions such as depression, anxiety and stress, as well as to fight off physical conditions such as obesity, diabetes and osteoporosis

brain is also responsible for muscle co-ordination and for the control of particular endocrine glands.

Exercise affects the nervous system by stimulating the activity of the chemicals which transmit impulses from one nerve cell to another. These chemicals are called neurotransmitters and are linked to changes in mood.

Research has shown that exercise can improve mood, and many people exercise regularly simply because it makes them feel good. This has been mainly attributed to the feel-good hormones called endorphins, produced by the brain and the pituitary and released during added stress to the body. They have a 'morphine-type' effect, producing the 'aerobic high'. It is possible to become addicted to exercise in the quest of achieving this high, and you should be aware of this in order to avoid possible 'burn out' and injury to joints and muscles. As well as stimulating endorphin release, exercise also uses up excess stress hormones, such as cortisol, which increases the feeling of wellbeing.

Exercise intensity affects mood according to the fitness of the exerciser. Activities that are too high in intensity for the exerciser can cause a negative mood swing because of increased tension and fatigue. Positive mood swings are associated with lower intensity exercise: about 60 per cent of maximum heart rate. Each body type needs to be aware of the intensity of their workout as this can influence their mood and their attitude and commitment to exercise.

It is not only aerobic exercise that promotes good feelings. Other forms of exercise such as yoga, t'ai chi, weight training and even relaxation methods can put you more in tune with yourself. In addition to aerobic work, these types of exercise have been associated with increased alpha waves, electrical patterns of brain activity which show that the mind is relaxed. Exercise is said to increase these brain waves, promoting a more relaxed state.

Taking a mindful approach to exercise is essential to all body types to ensure consistency and effectiveness in each workout. You will learn to draw upon sources of energy and inspiration to help you achieve your goals. If you have not worked out before, you need to focus your mind on your muscles, to ensure good technique and control.

Try the following test.

In kneeling or standing position with good posture and arms down by your side. Make a fist with your hands. Raise your arms in front of you to shoulder level then release. Now do the same thing and imagine you are lifting a heavy chain out in front of you. In order to raise the imaginary chain you have will have to concentrate on creating tension in your muscles. Focusing your mind on your muscles to create tension and give added resistance to a movement has the effect of working your muscles much harder than if you had just lifted your arms up and down.

BE YOUR OWN PERSONAL TRAINER

You can also help yourself by becoming your own personal trainer. Personal trainers are in demand because they encourage clients to work harder than they would normally do. They also constantly enforce good technique and posture. You can be your own trainer by focusing your mind to your muscles, concentrating on good form, and reinforcing teaching points and positive thoughts to push yourself to do those extra few reps.

Affirmations

Affirmations are positive statements that you repeat to yourself over and over again to change a bad habit and make a new good one, or to give yourself inspiration to boost your confidence and raise your esteem. It is said to take around twenty-one days to make a habit. If you start off using affirmations, constantly reinforcing correct technique and saying to yourself words of encouragement, you can probably build up good exercise habits for life.

Here are some examples of affirmations:

My muscles are strong and powerful
My muscles are becoming more toned and tighter every time I exercise
I am confident, relaxed and capable of achieving my goals

Visualisation

Fast becoming a popular way of ensuring goal achievement is creating mental images, or visualisation. This technique is used by many top athletes to enhance performance and it is very effective in motivation.

Before attempting visualisation it is important for each body type to be realistic about what they can achieve. It is no good our P-type trying to visualise being a T-type. Each body type must visualise themselves to be the best that they can be *within their type*.

If you like, start by visualising small goals, such as a small amount of weight loss, the joy of getting into a skirt that has been too tight, or attempting five extra press-ups and succeeding. The key is to be as detailed as possible. Bring in sensations and feelings as well as pictures. Visualise yourself exercising confidently with perfect form. Run and re-run the visualisation through your mind, imagining the feeling of your muscles contracting and tightening, bringing you closer to your goal.

It is good to clear out the stresses and strains of everyday life before exercising. Relax your body and your mind will relax too. Before a session, sit or lie in a comfortable space and breathe deeply, using the whole of your lungs to fill every cell of your body, not just the top half, with oxygen. Breathe in through the nose and out through the nose, and as you do so feel the ribs lifting outwards and gently falling again. Don't hold your breath or huff and puff or put strain on your abdomen by pushing it forward. Spend a few minutes breathing and focusing your mind on the workout ahead, visualising and reaffirming your goal.

As you start to exercise visualise yourself working with good form. Remember to put mind to muscle and make the most out of every contraction. At the end of your session, during your cool down or for a few minutes afterwards, focus on your breathing and praise yourself for the hard work that you have done. Acknowledge that you are one step closer to your goal of being the perfect shape within your type.

I wish you every success in the Apples and Pears fitness programme. Good luck, and be the best that you can be!

BIBLIOGRAPHY

Abravenel, *Body Type, Diet and Lifetime Nutrition Plan*
(Bantam 1983)

Ganong, *Review of Medical Physiology* (Lange Medical
Publications 1982)

Malina, Buchard, *Growth, Maturation and Physical Activity*
(Human Kinetics 1991)

Roche, Heymsfield, Lohman, *Human Body Composition*
(Human Kinetics 1996)

Wilmore, Costill, *Physiology of Sport and Exercise*
(Human Kinetics 1994)

ACKNOWLEDGEMENTS

My grateful thanks go to Mark O'Matthews at the Reve
Pavilion in Guildford, Surrey; Dr Dominic McHugh, consultant
surgeon Kings College Hospital London, and Joy Walters Grad.
Dip. Phys. (NZ), NCSP, SRP, MACP, Chartered Physiotherapist,
for expert advice. My thanks also to the Institute of Optimum
Nutrition for allowing me to sit in on lectures on metabolic
body typing.

I would also like to say a heartfelt thank you to Nicholas
Rees, my dearest friend, for his never-ending support and
friendship in this, the writing of my first book; and to Eve
Cameron, Sarah Clennel and Philippa Williams again for their
support and friendship. Lastly, I would like to thank my son
Jamie Thomas, for his patience in putting up with a mum who
is always working.